HOMEMADE SANITIZERS

A complete Guide to making 20 Hand Sanitizer Gel recipes at home.

Content Copyright © 2020 Sly Soave. All rights held. Any unauthorized duplication in entire or partially or dissemination of this release using any means (including yet not constrained to photocopying, electronic gadgets, digital forms, and the Internet) will be summoned to the furthest reaches of the law.

NOTE TO READERS: This book has been written and published strictly for informational purposes. The author and publisher are providing you with information in this work so that you can have the knowledge and can choose, at your own risk, to act on that knowledge. The views and opinions expressed in this book are solely those of the authors.

This book is independently authored and distributed, and no sponsorship or endorsement of this book by and no alliance with any trademarked brands or different items referenced within are guaranteed or recommended. All trademarks that show up in this book have a place with the owner and are used here for informational purposes only.

Table Of Contents

Chapter One - Introduction To Hand Sanitizers 1

Chapter Two - Soap Making 25

Chapter Three - Liquid Soap 55

Chapter Four - Liquid Soap Making 79

Chapter Five - Disinfecting Wipes 130

Chapter One - Introduction to Hand Sanitizers

Present-day society has seen a blast in wellbeing cognizant, environmentally mindful people. However, one essential component of overall prosperity frequently is disregarded: our homes. A large number of products we use to keep our homes clean are harmful to the environment and our families. Advertisers would have us accept that, to clean the correct way, we should buy an array of expensive products. This isn't valid. Making cleaning supplies with natural ingredients isn't just conceivable; it very well may be accomplished for significantly less money than you would pay for commercial products in the store. And keeping in mind that created everything without any preparation may appear to be daunting. I want to assist you in finding that creating your disinfectants is entirely pure.

Disinfectants contain antimicrobial agents, for example, pine oil, sodium hypochlorite, quaternary ammonium mixes, or phenols, which kill microscopic organisms and infections on surfaces. A surface ought to be liberated from overwhelming soil for powerful sterilization. Disinfectant cleaners contain surfactants and manufacturers to evacuate soil, notwithstanding antimicrobial agents to kill germs.

Disinfectants are products whose significant capacity is to kill microscopic organisms on a surface, however, which are not really planned to expel dirt, stains, or different soils.

Some commercial hand sanitizer contains ingredients as unnerving as the germs they shield you from, so why not make your own hand sanitizer from ingredients you select? This is an astounding venture for kids just as grown-ups since the undertaking can be extended to incorporate a conversation about cleanliness and cleansing.

You will set aside money, shield yourself from germs, and can alter the fragrance of the hand sanitizer, so it doesn't smell medicinal.

WHY HAND SANITIZER?

A great deal of inquiries has been posed several times about why we have to make our high-quality sanitizers. Before you consider making your high-quality sanitizer, here is the thing that you have to know first. Research shows that rapidly spreading an ethanol-based hand sanitizer onto your hands most likely won't kill those cold and flu bugs. The explanation, as per the examination, is because your fingers are as yet wet with bodily liquid.

Hand sanitizers can diminish the number of microorganisms on the hands, yet they don't dispose of a wide range of germs. Alcohol-based products show up as the best at decreasing microorganisms whenever used appropriately; however, many don't use a vast enough sum or wipe it off before it has dried.

The products can be less viable if hands are dirty or oily and may not remove synthetic substances, including pesticides and overwhelming metals. It should just be used, notwithstanding legitimate hand washing. However, the individuals who do use sanitizers are encouraged to be sure they're picking an item with at any rate 60 percent alcohol. Research shows that products with 60 to 95 percent concentration are more viable than lower ratios, or non-alcohol-based sanitizers.

These days, several maladies can be transferred by skin contact. If peradventure that you know about N1H1, you most likely understand what I'm saying. Be that as it may, we can't refrain ourselves or our kids from holding and contacting objects found in public places, where germs, for the most part, are found. So playing it safe is not a terrible thing. Washing your hands with soap and better is the ideal approach to keep the germs under control. Yet, as we as a whole know, it isn't constantly conceivable. Any place we go, especially when we are with the family, it is smarter to bring hand sanitizer to clean our hands at whatever point we don't approach soap and water.

There are numerous sorts of hand sanitizer products you can discover in the market. The best are those with 60-80% alcohol concentration as they are successful in purifying purposes and killing germs. Or then again, you can likewise go for the natural oil base sanitizer with disinfectant properties. Cedarwood, clove, lavender, lemon, pine, tea tree, and fundamental oils have clean and disinfectant properties. In any case, among these oils, tea tree oil is the most impressive because it additionally contains antiviral against parasitic and antibacterial properties.

There are a few distinct kinds of natural hand sanitizers accessible — or a crafty individual could even make her natural hand sanitizer. Every natural hand sanitizer has an antimicrobial fixing and a saturating fixing; ingredients could conceivably incorporate alcohol. These sanitizers are additionally accessible in different structures, for example, spritzers, gels, or wipes.

Numerous natural and even natural oils contain antimicrobial properties. These oils are essential in a conventional natural hand sanitizer. Some well-known instances of oils that are viewed as antimicrobials incorporate thyme oil, lemon oil, orange oil, and lavender oil. At the point when these oils, either independently or in a mix, are blended in with water, Aloe Vera, or another substance, they are prompt to kill numerous germs that cause ailment.

More often than not, a natural hand sanitizer will have to fix to saturate the hands. For instance, Aloe Vera, jojoba oil, nutrient E, and wood cellulose are on the whole natural ingredients that may mollify and alleviate troubled skin. A few components, for example, Aloe Vera, might be used as the base of the sanitizer. Therefore, when the antimicrobial oil is mixed with the Aloe Vera, a natural hand sanitizer is made.

The broad discussion among numerous individuals is whether alcohol should be used in a hand sanitizer. Ethanol, an alcohol that is gotten from corn, is one of the most generally used alcohols. It will kill germs; yet, a few people dread that small kids might be overexposed to alcohol from hand sanitizers. Others accept that its utilization may make a superbug that is impervious to drugs. Some commercially available natural hand sanitizers contain alcohol, others don't.

A natural hand sanitizer may likewise differ in its structure. For instance, some sanitizers are gels, while others are water-based spritzers. An individual could also buy a sanitizer that is as a wipe or a sodden toilette. While the gels and spritzers may keep going quite a while, the wipes are increasingly compact and can without much of a stretch be taken in high-germ zones, for example, on aircraft.

As a rule, an excellent natural sanitizer is one without synthetic substances. Therefore, it will be better for the client and better for the environment.

Whatever you pick, it is significant that the sanitizer has a cream to shield your hands and skin from drying. Presently, if you need to ensure the hand sanitizer you and your family will use, you can decide to make your hand sanitizer. It will set aside your money; also, you can by and by picking the ingredients to use.

Here are a few plans that you can use in making your homemade hand sanitizer:

Alcohol-based Hand Sanitizer

- 1/4 cup unadulterated Aloe Vera gel

- 1/4 cup grain alcohol
- 1/4 cup vitamin E
- 10 drops fundamental oils (contingent upon your inclinations)

All-Natural Alcohol-Free Hand Sanitizer Gel

- 1 cup unadulterated Aloe Vera gel
- 1/2 cup of vitamin E
- 1-2 teaspoons of witch hazel (include until the ideal consistency is derived)
- 8 drops of fundamental oils (contingent upon your inclinations)

Homemade cleaning products are protected to use when contrasted with those commercial ones that comprise of destructive substances and risky synthetic concoctions. Likewise, they are simpler to use and less expensive.

Here are a few recommendations that you can prepare yourself:

- **Air Freshener**

Of all the homemade cleaning products, air fresheners are the most needed. To battle that frightful scent, you can use vinegar, alkali, baking soda and lemon.

Lemons are ideal for killing awful scent in your home. You can hurl a cut of it in your processor to invalidate that stench in your kitchen. You can likewise sun-dry it and spot it inside your bureau to fend moths off.

Vinegar is well known for its stain evacuating characteristics, yet what many people don't know is that it tends to be used to invalidate and retain any terrible odour. Pour a quart of it in your platter and let it remain in your space for a few hours to get out any awful smell. You can likewise include a scramble of baking soda or a drop of lemon squeeze in it for most extreme outcomes, yet recollect not to blend each of the three so as not to try too hard.

Ammonia helps in killing smell, yet it likewise helps in releasing any tenacious dirt.

Baking soda is additionally immaculate due to its peeling properties. You can put it inside a crate; cut a little gap in it and leave in any restricted spaces in your home and let it work its air renewing enchantment.

- **Pots and Pans Cleaner**

Do you have those stains in your dish that you can't appear to remove using your customary soap? Baking soda is the appropriate response. Blend 1-3 spoons of baking soda with a quart of water and pour it in your pots or dish. Let it represent a couple of moments and flush it like you regularly would.

- **Floor covering Deodorizer**

It is the most straightforward of all the homemade cleaning products. Sprinkle baking soda on your rug before you start your vacuuming. Concerning an increasingly fragrant impact, blend cornstarch and bath powder with baking soda and once more, sprinkle it on your floor covering. Make a point to let it represent two or three hours before you begin vacuuming all together for its aroma to soak in.

- **Surface Sanitizer**

Regular scouring alcohol can be valuable for disinfecting phone collectors and other decision plastics, yet shouldn't something be said about those things that you use for keeping liquids or nourishment? A couple of squirts of lemon is the answer to your concern.

There are numerous myths and misinterpretations about hand sanitizers. Right now going to take a gander at certain realities to expose the myths and put any misinformation to rest.

One of the most mainstream misguided judgments is that hand sanitizers are practically faultless and that they can forestall the spread of every single infectious illness, including the cold or flu. Albeit a hand sanitizer can kill more than 60 percent of flu infections on your hand, the vast majority contract flu from airborne agents, by taking in the germs.

So regardless of whether you have used a disinfecting item, and your hands are spotless and free from germs, you can still get the infection and spread them. A hand sanitizer may be an increasingly secure preventive system for gastrointestinal illnesses, as opposed to contaminations, for example, the cold or flu.

Another myth is that they are not as powerful as traditional hand washing with soap and water, in taking out germs from hands. It isn't valid. Washing with soap and water works betters if your hands are soiled, that is if you have dirt in your grasp. Notwithstanding, if your hands look clean yet ridden with germs, at that point, an alcohol-based hand sanitizer is a superior alternative because the alcohol is increasingly successful in killing the bacteria.

Another myth is that hand sanitizers lead to dry hands. These products contain emollients, which are synthetic compounds that diminish aggravation by securing and alleviating the skin. As illogical as it might appear, an alcohol-based hand sanitizer is, in reality, less brutal on the skin than soap and water. Research shows that washing the hands with soap and water may keep the hands dry. A hand sanitizer can keep hands wet through.

You can make quality and effective sanitizer at home. While homemade variations might be less expensive, most don't contain the suggested 60 percent alcohol content, which specialists concur is the ideal concentration to take out germs

In as much as the item contains 60 percent alcohol, a well-known brand will work similarly as subtle as an exceptional store product.

Gathering all the hand sanitizer realities, we can securely say that an alcohol-based sanitizer is the best way to kill germs in our grasp, however just as long as the item is used sparingly and mindfully.

An alcohol-based sanitizer isn't just ready to take out a more significant number of germs than soap and water but, it is gentler on skin whenever used adequately. Furthermore, when managed by a grown-up, this item can be useful for kids too.

While alcohol-based sanitizers have confronted analysis recently, principally because of the high alcohol concentration, specialists state that a portion of these feelings of dread is unwarranted. Alcohol isn't retained into the skin to any degree to warrant these feelings of fear. Indeed, even with over the top utilization, the degree of alcohol retention is innocuous, best case scenario. Alcohol may add to some sanitizer risks, however not to an incredible degree.

The argument against alcohol-based content possibly holds up if the products are used in such a manner that they were not supposed to be used. For instance, an alcohol-based hand sanitizer should not be swallowed. However, there have been a few cases where children and grown-ups have taken the liquid and fallen exceptionally sick.

A few producers have endeavored to address the public's anxiety over alcohol content and began making alcohol free variations as a more secure other option. These products depend on plant oils to kill germs; however, so far have not been as influential as alcohol-based hand sanitizers. Whenever used in the appropriate proportion, an alcohol-based hand sanitizer is not any more dangerous than an alcohol-free variation.

MAKE THE USE OF HAND SANITIZER A HABIT.

Recollect that old nursery rhyme that says' "spotless little hands are acceptable to see!"? Indeed, our hands are not little any longer. However, the unquestionably must be spotless constantly! We as a whole know the significance of washing our hands appropriately; however, when soap and water are not accessible, we go to our trusty hand sanitizer to accomplish the work. Hand sanitizers are gels that contain alcohol which intends to kill microscopic organisms and infections. Since alcohol can cause dryness, most brands presently contain lotions to limit skin dryness and disturbance.

As per a few investigations, the danger of spreading gastrointestinal and respiratory disease is diminished with the use of hand chemicals among families, so it's acceptable to convey one in your tote constantly.

Powerful Use of Hand Sanitizers

Spot a modest quantity, (about the size of your thumbnail) on the palm of your hand. Rub it over your whole hand and your nail beds. You would realize that you have not used enough if the gel dissipates in under fifteen seconds.

What to Watch Out For

The alcohol substance of hand chemicals might be as ethyl alcohol, ethanol or isopropanol. Regardless of which sort of alcohol is recorded, its concentration ought to be somewhere in the range of 60 and 95 percent. Anything short of 60 percent isn't sufficient to be a viable chemical. While the utilization of alcohol is normal, a few gatherings have supported keeping alcohol-based ones from youngsters. They may lick the gels off their mind, and this can cause alcohol harming!

This homemade sanitizer is incredible for all skin types. Recall, however, this isn't implied as a trade for soap and water. Probably, their utilization is just a reciprocal propensity. This chemical is best when used with constant hand-washing.

ALL NATURAL HAND SANITIZER

Ingredients:

- 1/4 cup witch hazel concentrate
- 1/4 cup Aloe Vera gel
- One teaspoon of vegetable glycerin
- One tablespoon of lemon juice or natural apple juice vinegar
- Ten drops tea tree oil

Directions:

1. Spot ingredients in a lidded glass container and shake to join.

2. Spread on your hands and massage into your skin..

3. Rinse with warm water.

HOW HAND SANITIZERS KILL BACTERIA

Ailment causing germs are available around all of you the time—one principle course of contamination for these pathogens in your hands. Your hands are continually contacting the environment around you, getting pathogens as they go, permitting these harmful substances to taint you or spread to other people. To forestall this, the Center for Disease Control and Prevention suggests the ordinary washing of your hands with soap and water.

Sadly, clean water and soap aren't always accessible. In these cases, the CDC prescribes using an alcohol-based hand sanitizer, which is equipped for killing most germs.

Dynamic Ingredients

Most hand sanitizers' active ingredients comprise of either ethanol or isopropanol, the two types of alcohol. Alcohol kills most germs on contact without making genuine mischief the skin tissue, which makes it a viable, dynamic element for hand sanitizers. Ethanol and isopropanol are sterilizers that kill germs by dissolving their essential proteins. This upsets the typical cell action of the bacterium, making it bite the dust.

Idle Ingredients

To help in the application, and increment the skin advantages of the item, hand sanitizers regularly use inert ingredients close by ethanol or isopropanol. For instance, humectants, for example, glycerin, function as saturating agents. Humectants draw dampness from the general environment and hold it near the skin. Thickening agents, for example, polyacrylic corrosive, may likewise be used to give hand sanitizers a gel-like surface, which helps in the application and spreading of the item on the hands. A fresher advancement close by sanitizers is the use of essential oils to help reduce the smell of alcohol while applying the item.

Bacterial cells, similar to some other cells, have a plasma/cell film that encases the various organelles. The film goes about as a hindrance between the inside of the bacterium and the outside environment. Any harm to the cell layer would open the conduits for bacterial demise. This is actually how hand sanitizers work. They break up/cut off the cell film first and afterwards proceed to denature the proteins inside the bacterial cells.

The Breaking Down Of the Cell Layer

The cell film of a bacterium is made out of phospholipids. Phospholipids are a class of lipids containing two hydrophobic (water-despising and non-polar) unsaturated fats toward one side, alluded to as 'tails', and a 'head' that is hydrophilic (water-adoring and polar) in nature. The phosphate bunch appended at the head makes it polar and hydrophilic. A glycerol atom usually consolidates the two sections.

The tails may be hydrophobic, yet they are likewise lipophilic (lipid-cherishing) in nature. Hand sanitizers misuse this lipophilic nature of the tails to deteriorate the cell layer due to the "like disintegrates like" rule. The non-polar tails disintegrate promptly in other non-polar mixes.

The natural solvents which are propanol or ethanol, used by sanitizers are amphiphilic mixes—implying that they contain both a hydrophilic part and a lipophilic (or hydrophobic) part. They are ace solvents and can break up both polar and non-polar mixes.

Consequently, when the ethanol particles in your grasp sanitizer interact with the cell layer, they bond with it and begin dissolving the lipophilic tail. The layer, in this manner, loses its necessary respectability and gets burst in a lot of better places, spilling out the cell guts. In itself, this would cause bacterial passing, as the phone organelles would overflow out. However, hand sanitizers make it a stride further by denaturing the phone proteins.

Denaturation of bacterial proteins

You have likely understood over and over that proteins are the way to life. Devastate the protein atoms, and the life of the living being will follow. Denaturation is the separation of protein particles by the use of external pressure. External pressure can be as radiation, warmth or concoction mixes, for example, a solid corrosive or base, a concentrated inorganic salt or a natural dissolvable. Isopropyl alcohol, ethanol and propanol are for the most part instances of natural solvents.

The structure of a protein assumes a conclusive job in choosing whether the atom can appropriately play out its capacities or not. Upsetting the protein structure in any size or way would render them useless and eventually lead to cell demise.

Hand sanitizers denature proteins by interfering with the hydrogen bonds in the auxiliary and tertiary protein structures. In the optional structure, hydrogen holding shows up among amide groups, while in a tertiary structure, hydrogen bonds framed are by the side chains.

In the wake of debilitating the cell film, alcohol atoms start surging in and breaking these hydrogen bonds. When the new relationships between the protein atoms and alcohol are shaped, the protein particles lose their structure and, subsequently, their usefulness. As effectively settled, without these proteins working, the bacterial cell stops to endure and rapidly bites the dust.

Along these lines, this is how hand sanitizers work, by first mellowing the protection divider (cell layer) of the bacterial cell and afterwards assaulting their important gems (proteins). Be that as it may, hand sanitizers don't generally work. Scientists have seen hand sanitizers as inadequate when the hands are noticeably dirty and less viable overall than washing hands with regular soap and water. In this way, the FDA prompts washing your hands using standard soap and water and possibly using hand sanitizers when those assets are not accessible.

Adequacy

Hand sanitizers within any event a 60 percent incorporation of alcohol are compelling in killing microscopic organisms, including the Streptococcus microbes, just as the microorganisms that cause tuberculosis (TB). Hand sanitizers are likewise powerful against contagious diseases, only as wrapped infections, for example, the usual cold and flu infections.

Homemade Hand Sanitizer Recipes and Ideas

Vinegar

You may not know this, yet vinegar has remarkable antibacterial properties. It's so incredible right now it kills 99 percent all things considered. As an additional worth, vinegar doesn't contaminate the environment, it's not harmful, and it's sheltered to eat. The last methods you can use it on youngsters and pets also, without the dread of them ingesting the sanitizer and getting wiped out.

You can use white vinegar for this reason. Store it in a little, travel-size shower container and take it with you any place you go. Splash abundantly on your hands, and rub them together until they're dry. You can likewise shake them. You needn't stress over the smell, since it will disseminate rapidly, leaving your hands' microscopic organisms free and scentless.

In any case, if you believe you despite everything can't stand the smell, including a couple of drops of lemon or lavender oil to veil the vinegar-like smell.

Aloe Vera

Ingredients

- Six ounces of water

- One teaspoon of Aloe Vera
- Two drops of cinnamon fundamental oil
- Two drops of clove oil
- Two drops rosemary
- Two drops eucalyptus oil.

You have to mix them all and pour the mixture in a showering bottle. Pour some on your hands at whatever point you feel the need and shake or pat dry.

Cautioning – some essential oils are incredibly intense and can cause rashes and disturbance when applied straightforwardly to the skin. Use Aloe Vera in a bountiful sum, as it alleviates the skin and forestalls these sicknesses. Aside from that, don't use all the oils in the recipe if you have touchy skin. Pick two of them and set up the invention using those. Since they all have a similar antimicrobial quality, it will get the job done.

Alcohol Infused Homemade Hand Sanitizer

Ingredients

- 66% of a cup of scouring alcohol or ethanol
- 33% of a cup of Aloe Vera gel – attempt to locate the natural sort since it has less added substances than the average kind and it's more advantageous. You can supplant the Aloe Vera gel with vegetable glycerin.
- Eight to ten drops of an organic oil based on your personal preference – thyme, clove, lavender, peppermint, cinnamon leaf.

- Pour all the ingredients in an earthenware or metal bowl, give them a decent whisk, and pipe them into an immaculate jug.

Directions

Use 60 percent alcohol, because this is the primary way it will have the option to battle germs. Additionally, if need be and you discover his mixture somewhat aggravating, don't abandon it. Instead, include some chamomile essential oil, which will adjust it out pleasantly.

Hydrogen Peroxide Homemade Hand Sanitizer

You have to make a three percent arrangement hydrogen peroxide. The concoction has been demonstrated productive against microbes since when it interacts with it, it oxides it. This procedure makes the microorganisms break down.

The mixture is effortless to make and significantly simpler to use. Nonetheless, if you plan on hefting it around with you as your throughout the day hand sanitizer, you should store it in a dull shaded container and away from any wellspring of light. Investing energy presented to daylight will oxidize it.

Splash it on your hands each time you feel the need, permit it to foam and them shake or pat dry.

Cautioning – kids may not be available to the stimulating impression that hydrogen peroxide triggers in the surface of the skin.

Tea Tree Oil

This bewildering substance is hostile to parasitic, antiviral, calming, and antibacterial. It amazingly affects microbes, altogether obliterating it.

To make this homemade hand sanitizer, you should mix up to ten drops of tea tree oil with one teaspoon of Castile oil. At the point when these two ingredients are wholly consolidated, you can pour them in six ounces of water. Give the holder a decent shake before each utilization.

Cautioning – tea tree oil is known to cause disturbances, should you include a lot of it into your homemade hand sanitizer. To adjust this impact, add a teaspoon of Aloe Vera gel or liquid vitamin E.

The Sweet Smelling Homemade Hand Sanitizer

Ingredients

- Five to ten drops of lavender organic oil – ensure it is untouched and natural.

- Thirty drops of tea tree essential oil which should be of 0.5 percent concentration.

- One tablespoon of witch hazel which you can mix with a similar measure of high-proof alcohol.

- Eight ounces of Aloe Vera gel which must be untouched and natural

A quarter teaspoon of vitamin E oil - you can mix with glycerin. This fixing will relax your hands and make the homemade hand sanitizer last longer without ruining. In this manner, don't skip it.

In a little glass or fired bowl, include all the essential oils, and the vitamin E. Whirl them around until they are mixed through. Include the witch hazel or alcohol if this is what you're using and mix once more. This whole creation should then be added to the Aloe Vera gel. Mix it well to guarantee they consolidate consummately.

Tip – Shake the splash bottle tenderly before each utilization. If accurately put away, this homemade hand sanitizer should last you a while.

One of the few reasons why this recipe calls for lavender oil is for it to veil the tea tree oil's robust smell. If you don't care for it or think that it is oppressive, supplant the lavender with whatever other fundamental oil which you discover satisfying. Some significant decisions are savvy, peppermint, sandalwood, and rosemary.

Since this hand sanitizer has a determination of fundamental oils, you should test it out before genuine use. Give it a shot a little fix of skin and perceive how you respond to it. Remember about the remainder of your relatives who may be using it. They could build up a hypersensitivity too.

The 'No-Germs Allowed' Homemade Hand Sanitizer

Ingredients

- One cup of water

- A large portion of a cup of Aloe Vera concentrate – be cautious, since this recipe doesn't care for different ones. Rather than the exemplary Aloe Vera gel, it calls for focus, because the gel doesn't mix also.

- A quarter cup of olive oil - you can mix with jojoba, avocado or almond oil.

- 15 drops of tea tree oil

- 20 drops of essential orange oil.

Mix all the ingredients and make a flawless, orange-scented homemade hand sanitizer. If you are not very enamored with this smell, swap if for another, as per your inclinations.

Peppermint Homemade Hand Sanitizer

Ingredients

- 12 drops of lavender oil
- Six drops of peppermint oil
- Three ounces of Aloe Vera gel
- One ounce of grain alcohol
- One capsule of Vitamin E

The initial step of this recipe calls for you to mix the oils and alcohol. When they have mixed thoroughly, you can include the Aloe Vera gel. At the point when you're prepared, empty the whole mixture into a spotless and dry jug. You can use a splashing one or a plastic press type, similar to the ones you can find in stores.

Given the way that peppermint is a dangerous, potent essential oil, its ideal on the off chance that you don't use it on youngsters younger than six. Their skin is very touchy, and the oil may create them a consuming uproar, rashes, and disturbances. You can modify the recipe for this homemade hand sanitizer for **kids** as follows.

- 25 drops of lavender oil
- Three ounces of Aloe Vera gel
- One-ounce grain alcohol
- One capsule of Vitamin E or 400 IUs

Tips

– don't take it off before it has dried totally. It's the best way to ensure it's productive against germs and microscopic organisms.

– don't contact your eyes or your mouth following you've applied the hand sanitizer.

– don't use the homemade hand sanitizer on your reproductive organs

– If your hands are exceptionally dirty or oily, the sanitizer may not fill in as productively.

The Cinnamon Homemade Hand Sanitizer

Ingredients

- Four ounces of Aloe Vera gel
- Four ounces of 40 percent alcohol
- 20 drops natural clove bud essential oil
- 17 drops lemon oil
- Ten drops cinnamon leaf essential oil – ensure you use cinnamon leaf oil for this recipe, instead of the more conventional cinnamon bark one. The last is far more grounded than the previous and, even though it is better in case you're devising a diffusing mix or splash, it can bother your skin. Similarly, in case you're anticipating using this homemade hand sanitizer on youngsters beneath the age of six, forget about the cinnamon oil. With regards to little children and infants, you should attempt to dodge every single essential oil.

- Seven drops of eucalyptus oil

- Five drops of rosemary essential oil, natural

The premise of this homemade hand sanitizer is the alcohol. Gradually pour all the drops of oil into it. Tally them all cautiously, so as not to commit any errors. Shake the compartment as you go. Include the Aloe Vera gel and give it one final shake.

Tip – you can supplant the alcohol with witch hazel.

Witch hazel is a shrub, generally decorative, that develops in America and Asia. It likewise has some medicinal purposes, for which individuals use its bark, leaves, and twigs. To the extent the torments for which it very well may be used, witch hazel is useful for the accompanying.

Hemorrhoids – You can use witch hazel water as a help for the tingling, aggravation, uneasiness, and consuming brought about by hemorrhoids, just as other butt-centric conditions.

Little bleedings – similar water, got from either the plant's leaves, bark or twigs can stop minor bleedings.

Disturbances at skin level – Researches have indicated that the unique witch hazel balm called Hametum can mitigate skin aggravations, as long as they are mellow ones.

Although it is a remarkable, valuable plant that individuals regularly use for some, conditions, including for homemade hand sanitizer recipes, witch hazel can have some symptoms.

Stomach upset – whenever alcoholic or in any case ingested.

Liver issues – when taken in an enormous portion

Cancer-causing trigger – the shrub has a compound in its organization called safrole that may cause malignancy whenever taken in tremendous amounts or for an all-inclusive time.

Although there have been no convincing investigations, its best that pregnant and nursing women avoid witch hazel, for security reasons.

Gel Hand Sanitizer

Ingredients:

- 1 Tablespoon of Witch Hazel
- 8 ounces of 100% unadulterated Aloe Vera gel
- 1/4 teaspoon of Vitamin E oil
- 10 drops of Tea Tree essential oil

How can it work?

Witch Hazel – Witch Hazel concentrate is an all-natural item with astringent, sterile, mitigating, antimicrobial, antibacterial, antifungal, and sedative properties. You can peruse progressively about witch hazel uses and advantages. Those properties make Witch Hazel ideal for use as a hand sanitizer.

Aloe Vera – The gel from the Aloe Vera plant is naturally saturating. Its utilization close by sanitizer helps keep your hands delicate as opposed to drying it out. You need 100% Aloe Vera Gel – not the green or blue kind.

Lavender Oil – This organic oil is likewise a germ-free, antibacterial and antimicrobial. Besides, it makes stuff smell wonderful. You can discover Lavender Oil here.

Vitamin E – The expansion of vitamin E should help keep the item steady.

Antibacterial Hand Gel

Put this hand gel in your office, workspace, or homeroom. Squirt on varying and rub into your hand. One squirt is all you need.

The recipe takes a couple of ingredients and a brief period to make. It is sans alcohol as well!

Lavender and tea tree fundamental oils are the stars right now sanitizer gel. Both are notable for their antibacterial properties—and impeccably natural approach to annihilate undesirable microscopic organisms.

Essential Oil Hand Gel

Ingredients:

- 1 cup Aloe Vera Gel
- 24 drops of Tea Tree Essential Oil
- 24 drops of Lavender Essential Oil
- 8 oz Glass Pump Bottle

Directions:

Using a pipe, include all ingredients into the glass bottle, shake to mix. Name your hand gel. Make sure to stir a long time before using, or you can use soluble to enable the essential oils to scatter into the aloe better.

It is ideal for making a new jug of this sans alcohol hand chemical at regular intervals. There are no additives right now Aloe Vera gel is a water-based fixing.

Recipe at 1% weakening.

Essential Oil Gel Recipe

Tips

- When using essential oils on the skin, make sure to use just high caliber

- Lavender and tea tree essential oils are a fantastic decision for this recipe; you could switch up the fundamental oils to make various mixes for your hand gel. If your preferred oil organization has a disinfectant mix, you could use 48 drops of that original oil mix rather than lavender and tea tree.

- When purchasing Aloe Vera gel, it is ideal for searching for a natural and untouched gel, taking a gander at ingredients and see if what it is tight where it counts.

Chapter Two - SOAP MAKING

What is Soap?

Before digging into the craft of soap making, we should initially see precisely. What is soap? A few people tend to skip sections, for example, this and make a plunge directly into the course, giving a segment of things. Be advised that skipping ahead to find out about what you have to accumulate to form your first group may be harmful. To make something, one must comprehend the basics to be fruitful. Since soap making is so logically based. When you understand the standards and hypotheses about how soap is framed, and why it shaped, you will have the option to apply your learning not just to follow a recipe but making your own unique and cunning show-stopper.

You are in front of the game if you at any point took a science class, so put on. Your sterile garment and read on.

In its most fundamental structure, soap is the salt of a fatty acid. Actually no, not the sort of salt that we keep on our tables to sprinkle on food. A salt is anything that is the result of an acid and a soluble base responding. The sort of salt shaped from this response is subject to the quality of acid and salt that is joining.

Review from science, using the pH or potential Hydrogen scale, on this scale water is nonpartisan at a 7. Anything short of 7 is an acid. Anything over 7 is a soluble base. At that point, the scale permits soluble bases and acids to depict as solid or frail substances. More grounded acids tend to consume though more grounded soluble plates tend to corrode. The pH scale likewise gives us a perspective to test elements to guarantee that they are protected from being contacted or ingested.

With regards to soap, the acid that is used for the most part comes as fatty acids gotten from creatures and plants. Every fatty acid has one hydrogen, two oxygen and one carbon particle and has a carboxylic acid gathering hanging out toward the end. This carboxylic acid gathering comprises hydrogen and carbon particles. Presently, when fatty acids meet up, they connect themselves into groups of three and structure what is called triglyceride particles. The triglyceride atom joins to one particle of glycerin. Cling to that information while we change gears a piece.

A soluble base is a base that will kill an acid and break up in the water. At the point when a solvent base and an acid blend, the balance of the two happens through the creation of hydrogen and oxygen molecules during the response procedure. When soap initially began being made, cinders of plants filled in as the salt that was used to cause a response with the fatty acids. In these cutting edge times, soluble bases are made commercially. The antacid that is used, only, in soap making is lye.

Lye can be bought at a home improvement shop. It is otherwise called sodium hydroxide or then again burning soda. Lye is referred to as harsh on account of its inclination to be very destructive.

 Now we realize that soap is a salt that is made when a fatty acid is joined with an antacid. We understand what fatty acids and antacids are. Presently here comes the most significant soap making term you will ever learn. Submit it to memory. SAPONIFICATION. Saponification is the concoction procedure for making soap. Here is the thing that occurs in fundamental terms. The antacid works to part the fatty acids into two sections, fatty acids and glycerin. At that point the salt ties with the fatty acid. So once saponification has happened, we are left with a tablet of salt and glycerin.

You may now be pondering, so if we are left with salt and glycerin, how precisely does that make spotless things? Well, that is more science. At the point when soap joins with water, it goes about as a surfactant. A surfactant atom has oil solvent and dissolvable water parts. Along these lines, these atoms can encompass oil or dirt particles and carry them into the water so they can be washed away.

Alright. Since you have the entirety of that foundation data put away in your cerebrum, you are prepared to find out about how soaps are made. There are commonly four forms that can be used to make carefully assembled soap. You can decide to use the cold procedure, the hot process, the liquefy and pour strategy or the rebatching technique. Every one of these strategies will be clarified in detail as you read on. They all share something practically speaking in any case, and that is the saponification procedure that needs to happen at some point, some way or another to make soap. So you will consistently require oil or fat and a necessary (quite often lye) to make a conventional soap.

Soap Making Safety Guidelines

Security is in every case first. Working with Lye and prompting a synthetic response involves taking alert when endeavoring such systems.

Research about your ingredients to comprehend what you are going after.

Before you start, you must take as much time as is needed to comprehend your ingredients. For instance, Lye is a substance to be treated with care. Go through a few time finding a good pace with it, for example, if you spill lye arrangement, don't endeavor to kill it with vinegar. Instead, you have to wash it with overabundance water.

Regardless of whether it sprinkled in your eyes or mouth or on your skin, washing it with water is the main and best answer for evading skin or eye injury. If it spills on your clothes, remove the influenced clothes right away.

- **Follow your Recipe**

Concoction responses need to happen with a specific goal in mind. It is about extents. To an extreme or excessively little of something can bring about an unwanted impact. In soap making, all recipe ingredients are referenced by weight, regularly ounces as you use hints of every arrangement. This way, it would be extraordinary if you have your recipe printed-out so you can ensure it, rather than bobbling with the telephone or tablet while working with your ingredients, particularly lye, you may likely spill something. It might take you a few minutes to remember the recipe by heart, and afterwards, it would be a lot simpler.

The second thing you have to follow your recipes is a delicate scale. Get a decent quality kitchen scale or a digital scale. Ensure you test it out first with other weights, for example, a coin of weights to affirm your parity's exactness. When tried, you have to weigh out the entirety of your ingredients as per your recipe. It isn't encouraged to modify to transform anything at the outset.

A few recipes notice rates instead of weights which you can use to adjust methods as per your ideal amount yet in the first place. It is suitable for testing with a prewritten recipe.

- **Deal with Your Eyes**

Your eyes ought to be one of your primary wellbeing needs. A ton of things could turn out badly and enter your eye during soap making; in any case, you can defeat this issue by wearing wellbeing lab goggles. Lye or homemade soap or color powder all could discover their way at you, yet not on the off chance that you had wellbeing goggles on. You ought to never avoid this progression. You likewise need near to access to water to wash it if something goes wrong. If you need the most significant permeability, consider hostile to haze goggles.

- **Deal with your skin**

Much the same as your eyes, the equivalent is valid for your skin. Lye or homemade soap can be profoundly aggravation to your skin on the off chance that you were not wearing protective gloves. You can use latex gloves or elastic gloves. Dishwashing gloves are additionally excellent, yet they can be massive to work with. You could likewise secure your skin by wearing a cover or long-sleeved top with the goal that you don't have your skin uncovered.

- **Ventilate your Room**

It isn't prudent to work with a compound response and the raw soap smell with shut windows. Keep the windows opened in the room that you are in to inhale outside air.

- **Be Prepared for Spills**

Regardless of whether you wear defensive rigging, anything could occur. That is the reason it is continuously essential to have a plan B. Purchase a granular retentive or an all-inclusive permeable spill unit and have this close by. The spill could be oil, your soap, lye, and so on. Continuously keep a water supply nearby.

- **Ensure You Have Printed the Right Recipe Without Any Errors**

Now and again, individuals can compose anything on the Internet without having suitable information on the rates and counts. Ensure you get recipes from reliable sources.

- **Set up All Your Ingredients before Hand**

At the point when you start, there isn't at that point time to circumvent your kitchen gathering or to gauge the remainder of your ingredients. Keep everything prepared, and inside hands reach before you start.

- **Work with a Clear Space**

A mess is always a considerable impediment in any procedure. With heaps of messiness, the odds of blunder increment. Continuously keep an unmistakable working space.

- **Record Your Results and Learn from Your Mistakes**

It is critical to record the consequences of your groups with the goal that you can make sense of what turned out badly and keep away from it later on.

- **Fend Pets and Children Off**

- Name the Utensils You Used For Lye

Be mindful yet don't let that repress your inventiveness to diminish your fun.

The Soap Making Procedure

There are a few distinct techniques that can be used to make soap nowadays—the soap making process starts with mixing two separate apparatuses. The first is a mix of lye and water. The second is a mix of fats and oils. These two solutions are combined until a point called trace is come to. Trace is where enough saponification has happened that the blend has begun to thicken. As a rule, when trace happens, the soap has filled a form or some likeness thereof. Contingent upon the strategy for soap making being used, the soap will at that point experience a gel stage where it turns out to be progressively opaque in shading. A gel stage doesn't generally happen and doesn't fundamentally need to happen. At the point when a portion of the log form is used, the gel stage tends to occur because the blend holds its warmth well and will condense while in shape. Soaps that are filled in individual molds will not hold their heat accordingly and are not as prone to experience the gel stage. If the soap does experience a gel stage, saponification will in general be quicker. Regardless of whether it goes through a gel stage or not, after the soap has solidified in shape, it is taken out and put on racks to fix. The restoring procedure takes around three months and a half to complete and permits the soap to solidify and age. If restoring is finished, the soap is ready to use.

You may review from prior that the pot batch process is one way that organizations used to make extremely a lot of soap. Stated below is a four-step procedure which is straightforward.

1. Bubbling/Boiling

In this initial step, the fats and the antacid will be melted into a huge steel pot. Heat curls inside the pot heat the blend to boiling. Saponification starts as the fats and soluble base blend, delivering soap and glycerin.

2. Salting

In request to isolate the glycerin and soap, salt will be added to the blend. At the point when the salt has been included, the soap ascends to the highest point of the pot and glycerin settles to the base. The glycerin is removed through the base of the pot.

3. Solid change

A caustic arrangement is then added to the pot during what is called the solid change stage to remove any fats that have not saponified. This is imperative to accomplishing a soap that is smooth and free of debasements. The blend is boiled again, and the fat goes to soap. Salting can be rehashed now if essential.

4. Pitching

In this last stage, water is added to the pot, and the soap is brought to one more bubble. The blend will isolate into two layers after time. The top layer, containing about 70% soap and 30% water, is alluded to as "slick soap". The base later contains the rest of the water, dirt, and other debasements. This layer is called "nigre". The soap is shaped, cooled, and restored before it is wrapped and prepared for procurement.

The most current system used to mass-produce soap is the Continuous Procedure. It works this way:

1. **Splitting**

This initial step splits the fat being used to make the soap into fatty acids and glycerin. The procedure happens in a tall tempered steel section called a hydrolizer. Fat is siphoned into one end of the segment, and boiling water is siphoned into the opposite end. The portion is then profoundly pressurized. As the splitting procedure happens, the fatty acids and the glycerin are siphoned out of the segment while simultaneously progressively fat and water are added to the section. The removed fatty acids are then purged through a refining procedure to guarantee that they are smooth and liberated from contaminations.

2. **Blending**

A soluble base is presently blended in with the filtered fatty acids to create soap. Added substances, for example, shading, scent, and exfoliators, are placed into the blend during this progression.

3. **Cooling and Finishing**

The soap is filled shape and solidifies into a huge piece. Coolers are now and again used to accelerate this procedure. Bars of soap are then cut from the chunk and wrapped.

Since you have a decent foundation of what soap is and its history just as a fundamental comprehension of how it is made, the time has come to dive in more profound and get begun figuring out how to make your soap.

Equipment used for Soap making

Compared to many other crafts, you do not need much equipment to make soap and much of what you do need is inexpensive. In fact, you may as of now have quite a bit of what you need in your kitchen.

It is pivotal that once you use a device for soap making, you don't use it for cooking or some other action. A portion of the synthetics used in soap causing is noxious whenever ingested and can to consume the skin. Ensure you store your soap making utensils independently from your kitchen-use appliances.

While picking your devices, it is imperative to choose hardware that isn't made of aluminium, metal, or bronze when making soap. These metals respond contrarily to lye and will present security risks and won't produce generally excellent final products for your soap. Treated steel, glass, and veneer are acceptable decisions.

First here is a rundown of the nuts and bolts that don't require an excess of clarification:

- Freezer paper or saran wrap (not wax paper) to cover your work surface also, line the form if necessary

- 6-8 inch steel blade for cutting soap on the off chance that you are not using a form

- Drying rack to permit your soap to fix.

- Droppers or pipettes to include shading and aroma

- Rubber spatula to mix

- Stainless steel spoons to mix

- Stainless steel speed to blend

- Bowls

- 4-cup glass measure to guarantee you include the perfect ratio of each fixing

- Waterproof computerized thermometer ideally produced using hardened steel and at any rate 5 inches in length

- Rubbing alcohol in a shower bottle

- Crockpot (discretionary)

- Double heater (discretionary)

- Microwave (discretionary)

There are a couple of different bits of hardware you will require which require a piece more conversation with the end goal for you to have the option to settle on an informed decision at the store. The first of these things is a blender. You may conclude that hand blending works for you, especially on the off chance that you need to join soap making with your everyday exercise. Be that as it may, for some, blending soap for near an hour with the goal for it to completely start the saponification procedure won't prompt individual happiness. On the off chance that you are one of those individuals, you have two or three alternatives to consider. An electric hand blender can be used yet has its disadvantages. There is an inclination for a great deal of air to get included in the blend, using this method. This can cause some critical issues with the batch of soap, including have air pockets all through the completed item. The utilization of a stick or inundation blender is profoundly suggested. Search for one that has a straightforward structure with sharp edges that associate with the blender and a big part behind the sharp edges. You need to search for a low, short end on your mixer (around the edge territory). Likewise, discover a blender that has a smooth base edge. Abstain from picking one with sections or sides. Try not to stress about having a few speed settings; it won't make any difference as you will beat it or using it in the off position. By using a stick blender, you can chop down the time it takes to arrive at a follow altogether. We are talking from 45 minutes down to 5 hours.

Some soap recipes tend to isolate, and the danger of this happening is considerably less when using a stick blender. So now that the delights of the stick blender have been shared, there is a provision. You might need to mix by hand or on the other hand, use a customary electric hand blender when making your first couple of batches.

This will permit you to unmistakably observe the stages your soap is experiencing and, in specific, distinguish when you have arrived at the following organize. It is effortless to get a bogus follow when using a stick blender

Another significant bit of hardware is a scale. When estimating ingredients for a soap recipe, the estimations, especially lye and water, must be careful.

More careful than estimating cups would be without a doubt. Evaluating with a scale will make it almost sure that the soap making procedure will be sans glitch. It is moreover more secure as the synthetic compounds used will respond in a predictable manner that you have gotten ready for. At the point when you are buying a scale, you need to search for a few things. Right off the bat, you need it to be computerized, so you get careful readings. It will likewise, be valuable on the off chance that it can disclose to you loads in Metric and English estimations.

This will spare the way toward changing overestimations from recipes written in metric units into English terms and the other way around. Size is another thought.

You need your scale to have a useable surface of in any event six inches square. The scale's unit of graduation is essential. Soap making requires estimating some very modest quantities so search for a scale that measures in 1 gram and 1 ounce increases.

Since we are working with acids and bases that can be unsafe when they come in contact on the skin if not killed, it is advantageous to test the pH of your soap sooner or later. On a pH scale, numbers under 7 connote acids and numbers over 7 mean a soluble base. It is alluring for soap to have a pH of somewhere in the range of 7 and 10. Except if you purchase extremely costly lab-quality pH testing gear, you are left with two or three alternatives to test pH, none of which give us an amazingly precise perusing yet some data is better than no data.

The first, and most customary test, is to put a drop of soap on your tongue. On the off chance that it destroys like an electric stun, you realize that the lye has not been killed and you have to continue blending or cooking to bring the pH down and make the soap safe. The "hand test" can likewise be used. At the point when the soap is done, wash your hands with it. If it gives little foam and causes skin aggravation, the pH is likely not inside the protected range. If these thoughts are most certainly not speaking to you, travel to the drug store where you can buy pH strips.

To use these, put a drop of water on your soap and afterwards put the test strip on the water. Since this tests the pH of the water and not the hardened (or semi solidified) soap, it isn't exact, yet you do show signs of improvement thought of where the soap is at. Another device that can be used is phenolphthalein. This is a liquid that you drop in extremely modest quantities onto the soap. If the liquid is clear or light pink, you are good to go. On the off chance that it is a darker shading, you have to proceed with the saponification procedure to make it safe. Phenolphthalein is most effortlessly found at a store that sells pool supplies as it is likewise used to test the wellbeing of swimming water.

Soap molds are presumably the best time and intriguing bits of hardware you will search for. Soap molds come in all shapes and sizes. Some are very modest, and some are out and out expensive. There are a couple of general courses you can take to pick a shape. You could choose to buy singular molds to empty the soap straightforwardly into. Although those work very well for the soften and pour procedure, it doesn't turn out very too with the virus procedure as they are progressively hard to protect. You could likewise buy a wooden form called a soap portion or line a portion dish with cling wrap and use that (recollect not to use it for cooking after). When the soap as solidified, the soap can be removed from the shape and cut. There is an assortment of hardware alternatives for soap cutting. These include:

- Smooth sharp edge cutters

- Crinkle sharp edge shaper

- Single bar cutting box

- Soap edger

It's additionally simple to make your soap cutting box using a miter box. Here is how:

- Assemble materials

- Handsaw

- Ten 1-inch screws

- Screwdriver

- ½ inch by 4-inch poplar wood strips. Purchase enough length, so you have the range of your miter box times two in addition to eight inches.

- 1x2 inch wood strips. Purchase enough, so you have the length of your miter box times two in addition to eight inches.

- Wooden miter box

- Electric drill

- Cut two lengths of the poplar wood to a similar range as the miter box.

- Cut two lengths of the 1x2 blocks of wood strips to a similar range as the miter box.

- Three equitably spaced pilot gaps through the 1x2 strips.

- Drill openings in similar places halfway through the poplar strips.

- Screw the 1x2 and poplar strips together

- Spot the two side strips in the miter box

- Measure the opening between the different sides. This must be accurate as your end pieces need fit snuggly. This keeps soap from spilling out of shape.

- Cut the poplar and 1x2 strips to the estimation made in the last stride.

- Drill pilot openings and join the 1x2 wood strips to the poplar strips using screws.

- Put the pieces into the miter box.

You should take note that you can change the size of your shape by moving the end sorts further separated or closed out.

Your last shape choice is to get innovative and go insane. Here are some out of the case thoughts:

- PVC pipe

- Pringles can

- Cocoa can

- Silicone cake molds

- Candy molds

- Tupperware

- Shallow dish (you can remove singular shapes with dough shapers)

- Mini portion dish

- Tin can

- Box
- Yogurt compartments
- Fluted frozen yogurt dishes
- Muffin dish
- Margarine compartments
- Mail tubes
- Toilet paper rolls
- Paper towel rolls

If all else fails about whether an object can be used as a soap form or not, check the compartment to check whether it is dishwasher as well as microwave safe. On the off chance that it is, this is a decent marker than it very well may be used. Remember likewise that a form with one end more prominent than the other will discharge the soap all the more effectively after it is solidified.

If you are using a non-customary holder, it tends to be trying to make sense of exactly how much soap to make to fill it. Fortunately, there is a generally simple approach to discover this data.

1. Start by filling a shape with water and dumping the water into a liquid measure.

2. Measure the measure of water in ounces that the holder held and duplicate that by 1.8 (the quantity of cubic crawls in an ounce of water).

3. Duplicate this number by .40 to decide how a lot of soap oil you will need to place in the recipe to fill the compartment.

4. Duplicate that by the number of compartments you have.

5. Duplicate the measure of soap oils in ounces into the rates of oil in your recipe. For instance, on the off chance that you need 38 ounces of soap oils and your recipe calls for 35% olive oil, you will use 13.3 ounces of olive oil in your recipe (38 x .35).

Since you will use synthetics, lye specifically, the utilization of security gear is pivotal to forestall genuine injury. The accompanying wellbeing instruments are enthusiastically suggested:

- Safety goggles when using lye
- Rubber gloves when using lye
- Apron
- Vinegar and milk to kill lye spills
- Table covering, ideally one that can be discarded after each utilization (paper, plastic garbage pack, dollar store table fabric)

A large portion of the materials referenced right now be found by setting off to your neighborhood supermarket, home improvement shop, cooking store, or large box store. If you need to get extravagant with your molds, an outing to a specialty store, for example, Ben Franklin's, A.C. Moore, or Michaels would get you what you need. If you need to spare yourself from the problem of heading to a few spots, you can buy what you need quickly from the Internet. Most sites won't just sell hardware yet will likewise sell herbs, oils, flavors, scents, and bundling. If you are looking to make a lot of soap, there are sites where you can buy hardware and ingredients in mass, permitting you to spare a significant sum of money.

Soap ingredients

As you know, the significant ingredients that you will require to make soap are fats, oils, and lye. On the off chance that you need to take your soap up a score, you can include aroma, shading, or potentially herbs to make a vibrant bar.

Fats and oils

How about we spend a quality moment or two first. The fats and oils used in soap are otherwise called the soap base. The first alternative is to purchase fat from a butcher and render it yourself at home. Rendering is the way toward liquefying the fat and expelling any muscle tissue or different contaminations so you are left with a smooth material that won't ruin. The rendered fat from swine is called grease. This is a delicate, soft white substance. The rendered fat from sheep or dairy animals is called fat and is a hard, coarse strong. If you need to make your oil you will require:

- 3-5 pounds of fat that are cleaved (little) or ground
- Large pot
- Water
- Salt
- Sieve or Colander
- Large bowl
- Large spoons
- Potato mesher

When you have the entirety of your ingredients, set them out in a very much ventilated territory as rendering fat is an extremely foul procedure. If you have a side heater on your cookout, do this outside. The family will much be obliged. At the point when you are prepared to begin, follow these means:

- Put the little bits of fat into a significant pot and add only enough water to spread it.
- Include one tablespoon of salt for each pound of fat to the pot.

- Turn the warmth on and bring the blend up to a low bubble.

- Stew the fat on low warmth for 20-30 minutes.

- Use the potato mesher to push down the fat and accelerate the procedure a little by crushing more oil out.

- At the point when you are left with generally sautéed meat and cartilage in the pot, you can kill the warmth.

- Alert you should be exceptionally cautious while doing this following stage. Take the pot off the stove and pour the substance of the skillet through a colander or sifter and into an enormous bowl. This is best done in the sink.

- You will be left with all the solids in your colander and all the liquid in the bowl.

- Put the solids in a safe spot.

- Friend into the bowl and you will see a layer of water on the base and the dissolved fat on the top.

- Cool the liquid to room temperature and afterwards move it into the cooler to remain medium-term.

- In the morning, take the bowl out. You will see the grease or fat has framed a white plate on the water.

- Using a blade or fork, remove this plate and put the pieces into a bowl.

- Discard the remainder of the liquid. Remember that it might stop up your sink so dumping it into the fertilizer heap or the terrace is a smart thought.

- If that you made fat, clear off as a significant part of the free fat particles on it as you can. Run it under fresh water to ensure it is spotless.

- Store the grease or fat in the cooler until it is soap setting aside a few minutes.

If you are using animal fat doesn't sound engaging, it is splendidly satisfactory to use a vegetable base. This is normal, and an assortment of vegetable oils and shortenings can be found at the nearby essential food item or natural food store. Generally used soap bases are olive oil, Shea margarine, cocoa spread, and coconut oil. Olive oil is known for being delicate and is likely the most famous base. Shea margarine is exceptionally sensitive and ultra-saturating settling on it a decent decision for soap that will be used by somebody with dry skin. Using cocoa spread will add solidness to your soap. Coconut oil will create a hard soap with loads of air pockets in the foam at the point when it is used. Other, less healthy, fats and oils are jojoba, palm, sunflower, sweet almond, castor, chocolate, avocado, and cottonseed oil.

There is one final thing to know about as to fats and oils. At the point when you begin digging into recipes, you will see that some will allude to "super fatted" or on the other hand "super fatting" soap. This alludes to including extra bearer oil into your blend. Close to two additional tablespoons usually are added.

Lye

The following fixing that is required is a soluble base. Lye is an essential substance otherwise called caustic soda or sodium hydroxide. It is use for some reasons counting broiler purging, food restoring and channel opening. Be cautious when working with lye. It is a caustic substance truly equipped for consuming, eroding, or wrecking living tissue.

Lye can be bought at a tool shop. Be sure that what you buy is 100% sodium hydroxide or caustic soda. You may discover it with stove cleaners or Channel openers. It comes in a few structures including pieces, pellets, and micro beads.

What's more, coarse powder? Any of these can be used in the soap making process. Be that as it may; the most secure structure is believed to be pieces. On the off chance that you have hard water at your home, you might need to consider using filtered water when blending your lye for Better outcomes. Use care when using and putting away lye as it is harmful and Destructive.

Significant security note: Lye ought to be put away in clay, stoneware, glass, or heat-safe plastic compartments

Lotions

If you are hoping to make a genuinely saturating soap, there are a few ingredients you can add to achieve this. You may decide to include extra glycerin. Glycerin is a thick liquid that is lackluster and unscented. It is naturally delivered during the saponification of fats so you will have just made a few glycerin in your soap by joining fat and lye. Glycerin is a humectant implying that it sucks in and retains water from the air. This makes it incredible for keeping the skin saturated. It is water-dissolvable and has a low poisonous quality level.

Shea butter, coconut oil, almond oil, or nectar can likewise be included for extra moisturization. When looking for Shea butter, you will see that there are two types of accessible refined and grungy. Refined Shea butter has been handled at high warmth with synthetic concoctions. During that procedure, vast numbers of the advantages of Shea butter are lost. By using a foul Shea butter, you will procure the full profits by the item. If you decide to use nectar, include one tablespoon for each pound of oil and ensure it is completely blended in before the follow gets excessively thick.

Thickeners and hardeners

Contingent upon the kind of soap you are making and the structure components you are going to use to accomplish your ideal look, you may decide to include a material to thicken your soap or make it harder. There are a few decisions, the first of which is beeswax. This can be bought to make stores or stores that sell light making supplies. Beeswax enables the oils in the soap to mix and turn into progressively thick. By making a thicker base, the soap will balance out and become more earnestly.

Including salt will likewise build the soap's hardness, from the start. Observe that salt doesn't produce the hardness of the completed bar. However, it makes the bar get harder quicker. This permits the soap to be unmolded sooner. Salt ought to be broken up in the water before you add the lye to it. Use about ½ a teaspoon for each pound of oil or fat.

Water choices

Although it is generally reasonable to blend lye in with water when making soap, it is conceivable to use different liquids. Milk is here and there used in soap making to make exceptionally velvety soap. Cow's milk, goat's milk, coconut milk, and even buttermilk can be used. It is used rather than water in the lye arrangement. A note of alert Milk responds uniquely in contrast to water when blended in with lye because of the sugars that are in it. There is an inclination for the milk to singe as the lye warms up, and this could turn the blend darker and putrid (not positively). In order not to make this occur, the blending procedure can be altered a piece. This technique can likewise be followed to substitute tea, espresso, or brew for the water in the soap. It is critical to wear wellbeing goggles and gloves to do this.

- Start with 1/third of the milk in liquid-structure and the other 2/third of the milk in a slushy or solidified state.

- Set up an ice shower in your sink.

- Include the liquid 1/third of the milk to a tall pitcher or bowl.

- Spot the bowl in the cold sink water.

- Consolidate the lye with the milk, adding cold water to the sink to keep the temperatures down varying

- Gradually add lye to the milk and mix tenderly. Recollect that it is beginning to heat up now.

- Go incredibly, gradually permitting the blend to chill off a piece previously including more lye.

- Begin including the slushy or solidified milk to the blend. Be extremely cautious while doing this, so it doesn't sprinkle.

- Continue including, blending, and mixing until all the milk and lye has been consolidated. Try not to be frightened if the blend turns a brilliant golden shading. It will occur, and you should combine that into your overall soap structure when using milk.

Bubbles

Some portion of the enjoyment of soap is stirring up an incredible foam with vast amounts of bubbles. Two materials, borax and sugar, will assist you with accomplishing the objective of making extremely sudsy soap.

Borax won't just assist the soap make extremely incredible suds. It additionally fills in as a disinfectant. You can discover borax in stores, as a rule in the clothing soap segment.

By and large, one tablespoon of borax is used for each pound of soap base.

Sugar will likewise build the measure of foam and air pockets. One approach to include sugar to soap is to break down it in water before containing the lye completely. Another method is to take a touch of the water you have weighed for use in your lye arrangement and add ½ to one teaspoon of sugar for every pound of oil or fat. Disintegrate the sugar, using warm water may help with this. Include the arrangement when your soap is at the follow arrange before you include your scent. The last strategy for adding sugar is to make a syrup by consolidating two cups of sugar with one cup of water and gradually warming the blend. Mix until all the sugar is disintegrated.

Include 1/2 to one teaspoon of this straightforward syrup to your soap at following, before including aroma. Know that including sugar can expand the temperature of the soap during the gel procedure, so be extra cautious when dealing with.

Botanicals

Herbs and different botanicals are generally added to soap blends to give the soap mending properties, shading, or potentially scent. A few of these herbs can be developed in a nursery and dried. This is a reasonable method to get these fixings and is an excellent selling point if you are anticipating selling the soap that you make. If you have a nursery, plant a little segment of "soap botanicals" or Make a smaller than expected indoor nursery if you like. The accompanying botanicals are anything but difficult to develop and are extraordinary for using in soap making:

- Calendula
- Comfrey
- Lavender
- Mint
- Basil
- Rosemary
- Peppermint
- Spearmint
- Lemongrass
- Chamomile

- Sage

- Thyme

At the point when they are prepared, pick the botanicals and dry them before using it in a soap.

If developing herbs is excessive, head over to the supermarket or even better a regular nourishment store and buy herbs there. We will talk in more insight regarding botanicals later on right now.

Scent

Numerous individuals like a rank soap. There are heaps of alternatives, yet to the exclusion of everything else, try to pick added substances that are cosmetically protected, implying that they will not hurt skin. The rules for safe skin scent are administered by the Research Institute for Fragrance Materials and the International Fragrance Affiliation. While picking a scent for soap, you should choose if you are going to use scent oils or essential oils. Essential oils are the universal quintessence of a plant. Quintessence can emerge out of leaves, blossoms, bark, berries, roots, needles, seeds, beans, strips, cones, wood, stalks, or different pieces of the plant. A plant's embodiment is acquired either by refining or communicating it. One explanation fundamental oils are so costly is that it can take many pounds of plant material to make only one pound of essential oil. To make a pound of essential rose oil, it takes more than 2,000 pounds of flower petals. Know that even though fundamental oils are everyday items, they do contain usually happening synthetic substances that are not ok for the skin. Scent oils are falsely made aromas. They include synthetic concoctions, some natural plant or creature items, and manufactured fragrance.

The manufactured scent was created in the late 1800s and has become exceptionally well known. The two kinds of perfume will last around one year when putting away inside a dark glass in a dull, serene room.

Shading

Shading is a significant part of making soaps engaging and attractive to use. There are numerous sorts of muds, mineral shades, Micah, and flavors that are affirmed by the Food and Drug Administration for use in makeup. As with the aroma, you should pick a shading that is skin protected and endorsed for makeup. A few people mess with using colored pencils and kool help. Even though these are fruitful in giving your soap shading, they are not affirmed as being good your skin. Try not to use nourishment colorings, texture colors, light colors, paints, or pastels as these have not been confirmed for restorative use. Manufactured hues were found in the nineteenth century. These hues were called Tar Colors and were used in nourishment and beautifying agents. These synthetics were seen as destructive to people, and a significant number of them were prohibited.

Fundamental Techniques in making Bar Soap or Liquid Soap

Okay, you presently have the entirety of your hardware and fixings. It is currently time to choose which procedure of soap making you might want to use. Right now, you will figure out how each procedure functions and the advantages and downsides of each.

For a start, there are several things you should know for all systems. Significantly, you start by finding an all-around ventilated zone to work in.

When you discover, that spread your workspace. You can use towels, paper, or dispensable tablecloth. The reason for this is to secure the territory and take into account sheltered, simple cleanup. At that point, you have to put on elastic gloves and security goggles if you will be making a soap that uses lye. You should likewise have the entirety of your materials prepared first. The whole of the fixings ought to be estimated and in their proper holders before beginning to make the soap. Ensure all the fixings and gear you will require in later stages is good to go. In the event that important, line your molds. It is additionally fitting to peruse your formula altogether before you start. Ensure you comprehend the methodology you will be performing and the fixings just as the hardware you will use.

The remainder of this section will disclose to you a progression of procedures that can be used to make soap. The virus procedure, hot process, dissolve and pour, and rebatching systems will be canvassed top to bottom. Guidelines for how to create liquid soap and whipped soap will likewise be given.

The Cold Process

The primary ordinarily used method for making soap is using the virus procedure. The preferred position of the virus procedure is that there is a short 'dynamic' creation time (around 60 minutes). The soap made is typically increasingly smooth and even in surface than that created using different techniques. Because of the way that less lye is being used in this procedure contrasted and the hot methods, this kind of soap will, in general, be gentler on the skin. The impediment is that chilly handled cleaners need to fix for four to about a month and a half before using so the concoction change can finish.

The initial step is to make a water and lye blend. While picking your formula, it will determine how a lot of lye and how much water to consolidate. A decent general guideline if your recipe doesn't demonstrate a particular sum is to use 1-section lye, 3-section water proportion. It is critical to gauge the lye by weight and ideally measure it into a compartment that you can shut if you have to stop or your work is intruded.

Important security note: When joining, add the lye to the water and not water to the lye for security purposes. On the off chance that the water is added to lye, there will be a compound response, much like putting vinegar and heating soft drinks together. A holder that can withstand high temperatures must be used for blending because the substance response between the lye and the water will make the blend heat to around 200 degrees.

When the lye has been added to the water, mix consistently until the lye is disintegrated, or the required response won't happen when you blend this mix with the oil or fat. When joined, place a thermometer in the compartment and set it aside.

The subsequent advance is to set up your corrosive. If you are using a substantial fat, soften it to the liquid-structure. Measure your fats or oils into your soap container using a scale. Blend the fixings, put a thermometer in, and put in a safe spot.

This is the ideal opportunity to get both of your blends to a temperature of around 95 degrees. This is most effortlessly done by placing the lye compartment into cold water or an ice shower. You may likewise decide to warm your fat over the stove or in the microwave at little additions. At the point when they are both the necessary comparable temperature, empty the lye blend into the fat gradually while mixing. Significantly, you don't quit mixing until you come to the 'follow' stage. If you choose to hand blend, you ought to accomplish follow in around 45 minutes. If you use a stick blender, you can arrive at following in as meager as 2 minutes. When using a stick blender, you would prefer not to turn it on and let it get down to business. Instead, interchange beats with mixing movements while the blender is off. You realize you have the privilege consistency or have arrived at following when you can use your spoon to sprinkle a few of the substance on the rest, and it remains there for a piece before sinking. Remember that the time it takes to accomplish the following can fluctuate generally depending on temperature, mixing strategy, and sorts of fats used.

When the follow stage has been arrived at then aroma, shading, and whatever else you needed to include can be blended in. Join added substances totally and pour them into molds. Spread the molds with a top and enclose by 6-8 towels. No heat ought to escape as it is required for the saponification procedure to finish. Leave them to fix and cool for 18-36 hours.

Next, expel the soap from the molds. This is an ideal opportunity to cut on the off chance that you have chosen to make bar soaps. Spot the soaps on a cooling rack. Flip them each 6-8 days. The soap ought to be relieved entirely in 4 a month and a half. Encompassing the soap with outdoors and permitting it to solidify and age as the compound responses stop finishes this restoring procedure.

The Hot Process

Hot process soap is increasingly suggestive of prior occasions and of how soap would likely have been initially made. There are a few focal points and impediments to this method. The principal advantage is that you include fragrance; also, shading after the saponification process has happened in this way, changing their properties practically nothing. Hot processed soap is frequently somewhat gentler, making it simpler to cut. Then again, hot processed soap isn't too simple to form, and getting a smooth top layer is troublesome. Additionally, the process of cooking uses power and vitality assets not required by the cold process. It is conceivable to use a stove, double boiler, or Crockpot to make hot processed soap.

Similarly, as with the cold process, you need to make your lye and water mixture in one holder and your liquidized oils and fats in another pot. You don't need to hold up until they arrive at a specific temperature to join them when using this procedure. What you need to see when mixing them is partition. You would like to see yellowish curds on the last, a thick layer of oil in the center, and white foam on the top. When you see these layers, put the pot over low warmth and mix consistently (either by hand or with mixer). If you don't mix, the arrangement will boil over onto the stove or counter. This is risky and one of the reasons you are wearing security equip and have materials to tidy up lye close by.

Cook the soap until you get bubbles that are about the size of the leader of a pi. This should take around 15-25 minutes. Expel the soap from the warmth and let it cool until you don't perceive any air pockets, approximately 10 minutes. Warm on low until bubbles return. Cool again till bubbles are no more. Rehash this until no layers are left, and the mixture you have is even and uniform. It ought to help you to remember Vaseline. Include fragrance, shading, and some other wanted additives. Immerse your molds. There is no compelling reason to protect your molds as the saponification process has, as of now, happened. When the soap is cool, you can expel it from molds. If required right now is an ideal opportunity to cut the soap. Hot processed soap can provide a solution for as long as you feel vital. There is inconsistency among soap producers regardless of whether hot process soap should be restored at all while some remain by relieving for a month and a half. It is fitting to permit probably some relieving time with the soap on cooling racks.

Melt and Pour

The melt and pour technique is very popular with beginners. Using this technique is not soap making in real sense because there is no saponification process. Instead, glycerin is combined with surfactants to make a soap base that can be commercially purchased. Although this process does not require the scientific prowess that other methods do, it allows the soap maker to concentrate on the aesthetics of the soap, and the result can smell great and be truly beautiful. One of the significant benefits of this technique is being able to avoid the use of harsh chemicals such as lye. This is particularly desirous to soap makers with children or pets who frequently enter the soap making area. Using this technique is a great way to get children involved in soap making. To make liquefy and pour soap, start by softening your purchased soap base. This can be done in a microwave, Crockpot, or double boiler. Then, add any additives, colors, or fragrances you wish. Now pour the soap into your mold and let it harden. Once it's hard, take it out of the mold and let it dry on cooling racks for a couple of days before using it.

Rebatching

Rebatching, also called the hand-milled technique, is the last process of making solid soap that we will talk about. The benefits of this process are saving money and reducing waste from not-so-pretty batches of soap. It is also a way to revive old soap that has lost its scent. Since no raw chemicals are involved, children can help make this type of soap.

The first step in this technique involves making a plain soap using either the hot or cold process. Use soap to which no botanicals, dyes, or fragrances have been added. After the soap is hardened, grate it with a knife or cheese grater reserved for the purpose. Place the grated soap in a small heatproof container to microwave or put it into a mini Crockpot or a double boiler. Add nine ounces of water per twelve ounces of soap and melt it gently and gradually. It is essential when using this technique to work with small batches within small containers, so the soap does not burn. Do not allow the mixture to boil and be careful not to stir too much because suds and bubbles are likely to develop. Once the soap is melted, let it cool to around 150 degrees. At this point, add your botanicals, fragrances, colors, etc. Now it is ready to be poured into molds. When it is cooled, expel it from the molds. Slice, if necessary, and place on cooling racks for several days before storing.

Chapter Three - Liquid Soap

Some people prefer to have liquid soap for washing hands rather than a solid bar. Liquid soap also has the benefit of being ready to use in about 3 days instead of 3 weeks.

The first way to make liquid soap is to follow the recipe for a pure soap made with the cold process. Adhere to the directions as per the formula you want to use. Make sure it gets well beyond a trace before molding. Instead of curing your soap as directed, it will only sit for about three days then follow these steps:

- Remove the soap from the mold

- Shave, chop, or grate it. Make sure you use gloves for this process as the soap is still caustic.

- Mix 1 cup of the soap pieces with the chosen fragrances, dyes, etc.

- Put the combination in a double boiler or crockpot with 3 cups of water.

- Melt the soap gradually while stirring.

- Break up any clumps with a plastic whisk or fork. You may find that some pieces do not melt. If this is the case, you will need to strain the mixture later.

- Once the soap has melted to a point you think is appropriate, scoop some out and allow it to cool in a water bath. It should be runny when cooled.

- If it is excessively thick, you can include more water.

- If it isn't sufficiently thick, you can add extra soap pieces.

- Reheat as needed to get the right texture.

- Once you feel it's ready, strain the soap into a container.

The other method of making liquid soap involves an oven. The process is similar to making a hot process bar soap, except it uses a different type of lye.

Instead of using sodium hydroxide, liquid soap uses potassium hydroxide. To make hot process liquid soap, follow this procedure:

- Mix your lye-water solution and set it to cool (warning-potassium hydroxide will get hotter more quickly when mixed with water than sodium hydroxide).

- Mix your fats and oils.

- Blend the lye solution with the oils in an oven-safe pot until it reaches trace. This could take a while with liquid soap, but you will notice that when trace starts, the soap thickens very quickly

- Cover the pot with a cover that fits securely.

- Put the pot in a 180-degree oven.

- Cook for 4-5 hours, stirring every 20-30 minutes.

- When the soap is relatively clear, remove it from the oven.

- The paste now needs to be diluted. Bring 40 oz. of distilled water to a boil.

- Add the water to the soap.

- Stir it in.

- Put the top on the pot and pause for about an hour.

- Stir.

- Put the lid on overnight and stir again in the morning.

- Add fragrance and color.

-   Let rest.

- Store and enjoy.

Whipped soap

Whipped soap is a fun variation on the cold process of soap making. The result is whimsical soap resembling meringues, clouds, and puffs of whipped cream. To make whipped soap follow these steps:

1. Find a recipe with a percentage of hard oils (a.k.a. coconut, palm, lard, tallow, palm kernel, shea butter, cocoa butter, shortening) that is greater than 80%.

2. Weigh out your hard oils and place them in a glass mixing bowl.

3. Whip all of the oils with a hand mixer until peaks form.

4. Slowly add the liquid oils.

5. Whip for several minutes to achieve peaks again.

6. Add the lye-water solution your recipe calls for to the oils a couple of tablespoons at a time.

7. Keep whipping

8. And whip some more

9. Add fragrance, keeping in mind that this will decrease your peaks a bit.

10. Depending on the oils used, the soap will be done when it resembles thick yogurt, soft-serve ice cream, whipped butter, cream cheese, or whipped egg whites.

11. Add color.

12. Mold. Whipped soap works best in 'sliceable' molds. You can also use the soap to "frost" or pipe designs onto other prepared soaps as you would a cake or cookie.

13. Whipped soap will take at least 24 if not 36 hours to set.

14. Let it cure for several weeks.

Cleaning up

Now that your soap is made, it is time to clean up. Hopefully, you worked in an organized fashion, and no spills were making the cleanup process much more comfortable. When cleaning, remember that lye is now in several places, 2 pots and any tools that you used for mixing. It could also be on your gloves, the thermometer, and the scale. It is still unsafe and caustic because it did not have to opportunity to react with fat and saponify. Raw soap is acid, so be careful while cleaning up. The first step is to deal with leftover natural soap. Use a rubber spatula to scrape the soap out of your pot and into your molds; the less soap you have in your pot, the easier it will be to clean. Now rinse all of your containers and tools. Wipe your pot out with paper towels and dispose of them immediately. It is also possible to use "shop" towels, leave them out overnight before putting them in the wash so the saponification process from the leftover ingredients will complete, and no chemical reactions will occur in the washing machine. Alternatively, you can use a lot of hot water and "real" soap to wash the pot. You could also put all of your tools needing cleaning into the pot, cover it with a lid, and leave it overnight. By the next morning, the oils and lye that had remained will be soap. Just clean it up in the sink and dry. Do not wash your materials in your dishwasher; the reaction will cause water to spill out onto your floor.

Storing soap

After your soap has cured, an appropriate way to store it must be found. Keep in mind that the shelf life of homemade soap is much less than commercially made soap and becomes even shorter if it is not stored correctly. Homemade soap can last about a year when kept in a cool, dry spot. Placing it in an airtight container that is placed in a dark, dry, cool spot is ideal. Once you begin to use your soap, it is essential to keep it as dry as possible so that it lasts longer. Adding your dyes, botanicals, essences, and fragrances, cutting those shapes

Now that the basic soap mixture has been made, it's time to get creative with color, aroma, shapes, botanicals, and designs. The first part of this chapter will talk about fragrance options. We will then move onto coloring and then to botanicals. The chapter will end by outlining some design techniques to experiment with.

Scents

Being able to have a great smelling soap is one of the reasons to make your own. The point at which you add your fragrance varies depending on the method you used to make your soap. If the cold process was used, slowly add fragrance once the soap mixture is thoroughly blended, but before it begins to get too thick. You can play around with it, but you generally want to add between 5 and 7 ounces of fragrance per pound of fat/oil in the recipe. That's about 1-4 drops. With the melt and pour technique, fragrance oil should be added to your soap after the soap has been removed from the heat source and has had a chance to cool slightly. Use between 3 and 5 ounces of fragrance per pound of soap. If you add scent when the melted soap is too hot, it may "burn off." If you used the hot process, add the fragrance when the soap is the texture of meshed potatoes, right before it is poured into molds. As a side note, be aware that vanilla fragrances, or blends containing vanilla, are likely to turn your soap brown over time. This is fine, but you may want to consider that when choosing colors as you may want to add more browns, reds, or golds.

There are many options for fragrance. Choosing depends on several factors, including the user's skin type, gender, skin sensitivity, and desired benefits.

Many fragrances or materials added to provide fragrance have healing qualities and benefits beyond smelling good. Frequently, the scent is achieved by adding herbs or plants. Essential oils, straightforwardly from the plant, can also add their healing properties.

Here are several standard options and their benefits.

.

Ginger has a warm, spicy scent. It has antibacterial, antioxidant, and antiseptic properties. Ginger is thought to be beneficial for improving memory, decreasing muscular pain, and sharpening the senses. Its essence will provide the soap with a pale yellow color. Ginger may cause sensitivity in some people.

Anise has a robust and warm licorice scent. It has antiseptic and insect repelling properties. Anise is thought to be beneficial for relieving muscular aches and pains, coughs, and colds. It will provide the soap with a pale yellow color.

Fennel and a licorice scent. It is known to brighten dull skin, improve memory, and balance oily skin. Its essence will provide the soap with a pale yellow color.

Grapefruit has a fresh citrus scent. It is an antiseptic, antitoxic, and astringent. It is suitable for relieving acne, oily skin, depression, headaches, and also for toning skin. Its essence will provide the soap with a pale yellow color.

Lemon has a fresh citrus scent. It has antibiotic, antidepressant, antiseptic, astringent, and bug repelling properties. It is beneficial for treating acne, arthritis, colds, and depression, healing cuts, improving oily skin, reducing wrinkles, and strengthening fingernails.

Lemon essence will provide the soap with a pale yellow color. Lemon essence applied to the skin may cause sensitivity to light.

Sweet marjoram has a warm, spicy scent. It has antioxidant, antiseptic, antiviral, and antibacterial properties. Marjoram helps to relieve anxiety, headaches, bruising, colds, insomnia, and vertigo. Its essence will provide the soap with a pale yellow color.

Oregano has a strong, spicy, herbaceous scent. It has antiseptic, antitoxic, antiviral, bactericidal, fungicidal, and parasitic properties. It can be used to fight infections, relieve the itch, and treat athlete's foot.

Peppermint has a strong minty scent. It antidepressant, antiseptic, astringent, and insect repelling properties. Peppermint helps to treat acne, dermatitis, eczema, headaches, insect bites, migraines, and mental fatigue.

Its essence provides the soap with a pale yellow scent. This botanical may cause skin sensitivity.

Basil has a light, fresh, sweet herbaceous scent. It has antidepressant, antiseptic, anti-inflammatory, and antibacterial properties. Basil can fight fatigue, depression, wasp and mosquito bites, and headaches. Its essence will provide the soap with a pale yellow color. Basil may cause skin sensitivity.

Clary sage has an earthy scent. It has antiseptic, antidepressant, and aphrodisiac properties. It is beneficial to the treatment of acne, dandruff, depression, excessive perspiration, hair loss, inflamed skin, migraines, fatigue, anxiety, oily skin, and varicose veins. It also helps to promote sleep and reduce the appearance of wrinkles. Sage essence provides the soap with a golden yellow color.

Jasmine has a deep floral scent. It has antidepressant, anti-inflammatory, antiseptic, and aphrodisiac qualities. Jasmine helps relieve anxiety, depression, dry skin, and headaches. Its essence will provide the soap with a clear to pale yellow color.

Lemongrass has an earthy citrus scent. It has astringent, antiseptic, antifungal, anti-inflammatory, antidepressant, antiviral, fungicidal, bactericidal, and insect repelling properties. Lemongrass helps to treat oily skin, acne, headaches, athlete's foot, and excessive perspiration. Its essence provides the soap with a light yellow color.

Myrrh has a rich, earthy scent. It has antifungal, anti-inflammatory, antiseptic, antiviral, astringent, and sedative properties. Myrrh helps to treat athlete's foot, colds, cracked skin, and eczema. It can also sanitize cuts and decrease skin wrinkles. Its essence provides the soap with a dark brown color.

Rosemary has a deep herbaceous scent. It is helpful in cell renewal, reducing varicose veins, and stimulating hair growth. It cleans oily hair well.

Bergamot has a citrus scent with floral notes. It has antidepressant, antiseptic, deodorizing, and astringent properties. It is used to treat anxiety, depression, stress, fatigue, eczema, psoriasis, acne, insect bites, wounds, ulcers, and herpes. Bergamot essence will provide the soap with a greenish color.

Clove has a warm, spicy scent. It has antibiotic, antifungal, antioxidant, antiseptic, parasitic, and aphrodisiac properties. Clove helps to treat acne, athlete's foot, bruises, burns, infections, muscle pain, nausea, and warts. It can also be used as an insect repellant. The clove essence provides the soap with a golden color.

Geranium has a floral scent. It has astringent, antiseptic, antidepressant, antibiotic, and insecticidal properties. Geranium is helpful in treating eczema, dermatitis, psoriasis, acne, athlete's foot, bruises, burns, depression, lice, and pre-menstrual syndrome.

Juniper berry has a fresh pine scent. It has antiseptic and astringent properties. It helps treat acne, clogged pores, eczema, psoriasis, and inflammations. It is frequently used during meditation. Juniper berry essence will provide the soap with a clear to pale yellow color.

Lime has a strong citrus scent. It has astringent, antiseptic, antiviral, bactericidal, and deodorizing properties. Lime is beneficial for treating acne, arthritis, colds, infections, skin irritations, oily skin, and insect bites. It is also known to help strengthen nails.

Black pepper has a sharp, spicy scent. It has antimicrobial, antitoxic, antiseptic, bactericidal, and aphrodisiac qualities. Black pepper is known to help improve memory and reduce symptoms of colds, flu, and viruses. It can also help alleviate arthritis and other muscle aches and pains. Its essence will provide the soap with a light green color.

Eucalyptus has a strong herbaceous scent. It has antibiotic, antifungal, antiseptic, anti-parasitic, antiviral, decongestive, deodorizing, and stimulant properties. It is helpful in soothing bug bites, blisters, burns, rashes, chickenpox, and measles. Eucalyptus works as an insect repellant. It can help relieve nasal congestion, mental exhaustion, and muscle aches.

Lavender has a floral scent. It is used to relieve relieving depression, insomnia, headaches, nervous tension, and pain. Lavender has disinfecting properties and can help acne, eczema, and dandruff. Lavender essence will provide the soap with a light yellow color.

Orange has a light citrus scent. It has antiseptic, anti-inflammatory, antidepressant, fungicidal, and bactericidal properties. It is used to treat anxiety, oily skin, tension, and stress. Orange essence provides the soap with a light orange color. It can cause skin sensitivity in some.

Patchouli has a warm earthy scent. It has antibiotic, antidepressant, anti-infectious, anti-inflammatory, antifungal, antimicrobial, antiseptic, antiviral, aphrodisiac, astringent, bactericidal, and deodorizing properties.

Patchouli can help to treat acne, anxiety, athlete's foot, bacterial infections, cracked and chapped skin, dandruff, depression, dermatitis, dry skin, eczema, and fungal infections. Its essence provides the soap with a golden brown color.

Pine has a strong evergreen scent. It has antiseptic, antiviral, antibacterial, fungicidal, and deodorizing properties. Pine is used to treat excessive perspiration, eczema, psoriasis, lice, fleas, and mental fatigue. Its essence provides the soap with a pale yellow color. It can cause skin sensitivity for some people.

Sandalwood has a sweet, woodsy scent. It has antibacterial, antidepressant, antiseptic, aphrodisiac, astringent, emollient, fungicidal, insecticidal, and sedative properties. Sandalwood is beneficial for treating acne, anxiety, cracked and chapped skin, depression, dry skin, impotence, insomnia, nervous tension, scarring, and stress. Its essence provides the soap with an orange-brown color.

Ylang ylang has an earthy, spicy scent. It used for treating acne, insect bites, insomnia, and depression. Ylang-ylang essence provides the soap with a pale yellow to golden color. It can cause sensitivity for some people.

If you have trouble deciding on a single scent to use, feel free to stop stressing and blend several scents together. You will want to select at least 3 scents; a top note, middle note, and base note. The high note will be that first light scent that you detect but quickly fades. The middle note forms the majority of the scent and is the strongest and longest-lasting scent. The base note is rich and heavy; it will be the last scent detected but will linger. If this seems like too much for you, consider purchasing an already made fragrance blends. They are easily found and reasonably priced.

Color

Color is an essential aspect of making our soap look appealing and desirable to use. Synthetic colors have the advantage of providing very vibrant colors. FD & C colorants are very widely used in synthetical products. They come in a wide variety of colors, named by numbers, and can be purchased in powder and liquid forms. They have the benefit of being reasonable and are great for use in melt and pour soaps. FD and C colorings do not work as well in cold process soaps as they tend to be unstable and bleed. Using dyes will give your soap a lighter, transparent color.

Another form of coloring to choose from is pigment. These have been manufactured in laboratories since the 1970s. Pigments are inexpensive and work well in all types of soap making processes. They work particularly well for creating swirls, as they do not bleed. Mineral pigments include chromium compounds, Ferro cyanides, iron oxides, manganese compounds, titanium dioxide, and ultramarines. Using dyes will give your soap a more intense, full color.

Mica colorants will give the soap a shimmering effect. Not all micas are stable in cold and hot process soap making, so test a small amount before coloring the entire batch. They come in a wide variety of colors. Although mica itself is natural, coloring products usually have synthetic colorants added to them to provide a durable color coating. They are more expensive to use and require a more significant amount per batch. One way to use small amounts of Micah is to paint powdered Micah onto molded soap for some added texture and shimmer.

There are several types of natural colorants, including herbs, spices, and clays.

See below to get ideas on how to achieve your desired color using herbs and spices.

Yellow/Orange

- Turmeric
- Carrot
- Unrefined palm oil

- Cucumber
- Annatto seeds
- Calendula
- Tomato paste
- Powdered sun-dried tomato
- Paprika
- Rosehips and hawthorn
- Ginger essence
- Anise essence
- Fennel essence
- Grapefruit essence
- Lemon essence
- Marjoram essence
- Peppermint essence
- Juniper berry essence
- Lavender essence
- Orange essence
- Pine essence
- Ylang ylang essence
- Safflower powder

- Ground chamomile
- Curry powder
- Orange juice
- Pumpkin
- Saffron petals

Brown/Black

- Cocoa powder
- Coffee grounds
- Nutmeg
- Cinnamon
- Alkanet root
- Myrrh essence
- Rosehip seeds
- Vanilla essence
- Patchouli essence
- Sandalwood essence
- Dead sea mud
- Alkanet
- Coffee
- Black walnut hull

- Ground cloves
- Allspice
- Elderberries
- Olive leaf powder
- Ground pumice

Green

- Bentonite clay
- Pandan leaves
- Avocado
- Olive leaf with safflower powder
- Green stevia with safflower powder
- Green stevia with hawthorn
- Rosemary
- Bergamot essence
- Black pepper essence
- Burdock leaf
- Comfrey leaf
- Dandelion leaf
- French green clays
- Alfalfa

- Chamomile essential oil
- Chlorophyll
- Cucumber
- Green tea powder
- Ground henna
- Kelp
- Spearmint
- Spinach
- Wheatgrass juice
- Wood powder

Red/Pink

- Dried peppers
- Paprika
- Madder root
- Sandalwood powder
- Moroccan red clay
- Beetroot
- Cochineal powder
- Tree

Purple/Blue

- Alkanet
- Azulene
- Blue cornmeal
- Indigo root
- Rattanjot

Clays can be added to soap not only for color but for the properties they add to the soap as well. Kaolin is a white clay that adds a silky feel and creaminess to the soap. Rose clay will add a rose color and add a silkiness and absorbency to the finished soap. Rhassoul is a light brown clay that will give you a soap great for absorbing oils and impurities from the user's skin. A good rule of thumb is to add about 2 teaspoons of clay per pound of oil. Clays can be added to soap in several ways. It can be dissolved in the lye-water mixture. Alternatively, it can be added to the oil mixture. If you are looking to have the clay be swirled within the bar of soap, you can make a slurry out of oil and clay and add that to the mixture. This is accomplished by adding your lye-water mixture to your combined and melted oils. Do not mix too much before removing a cup or 2 of the concoction. Add the clay to the extracted lye-oil mixture. Stir the remainder of the lye and oil until it is almost ready to be poured into molds. At this point, add the clay slurry back into the pot to make a swirl. You could also swirl while in the mold, depending on your preference. To have the small and large mixtures reach trace at the same time, you are going to need to work quickly.

Once you choose your coloring agent, it is time to determine how much to add. A general rule is to add one tablespoon of a botanical colorant per pound of oils, but this can vary. If you are using a dye or pigment, start by adding ½ an ounce of color per ¾ of a pound of fat. Some colorings may need to be dissolved or incorporated into the liquid oil before being added to the larger batch. The result of coloring achieved from a particular medium can vary widely from recipe to recipe. Colorings are affected by which oils and fats are used, whether or not your soap goes through a gel process, how the dye reacts to lye, and also what fragrances are added. Most colorants are added at trace before molding when using the cold process soap making procedure.

When choosing your colorants and preparing to store your colored soap, keep in mind that many colorants are not lightfast. This means that when exposed to light, even artificial light, they will fade. Mineral pigments and Micah tend to be the most lightfast. This is yet another reason to store your soaps in a dark place.

Botanicals

Adding botanicals is a great way to increase the color, fragrance, and healing properties of your soap. Botanicals can be added in fresh or dried form. It is essential not to incorporate fruits and vegetables that have not to be preserved or dehydrated as they will cause your soap to spoil and go rancid very quickly.

Botanicals ground into a powder is added when the soap has reach trace. An oil infusion can also be made with the herbs.

Fresh flower petals are beautiful in soap. They work best with melt and pour soap. If they are added to cold process soap, they are likely to turn brown or black during the gel phase of the saponification process that occurs during curing. This does not mean you cannot use them; do not expect them tom look like the lovely petals you put in when the product is finished. There is one commonly available flower that will maintain its color after saponification and that is the calendula or pot marigold.

If you have grown fresh herbs that you would like to use, they need to be dried before being added to soap, so the soap does not spoil. One way to accomplish drying is by microwaving. This is the fastest method; however, it can cause the herbs to lose some healing properties. If this is the method you would like to try, use the following procedure:

- Place herbs on a piece of paper towel in a single layer.
- Cover the herbs with two more paper towels.
- Place in the microwave.
- Microwave for one minute.
- Check them.
- If they are still damp, microwave another minute.
- You may need to change the paper towels if they are wet or starting to burn.
- Continue until the herbs are dry.

Another way to dry herbs is by bundling. This is accomplished by:

- Gather the herbs in a small bunch.
- Tie the stems with a touch of twine, string, or yarn, keeping in mind not to tie so tightly that air cannot circulate within the bundle.
- Hang the herb bundles flower side down near a shady window.
- The herbs should be dry in one to two weeks.
- Store dried herbs in water/air proof holders away sunlight.

The last common way of drying herbs is by using the oven. Here is the procedure:

- Lay herbs on a cookie sheet in a single layer.
- Place on top of the stove.

- Heat your oven up to 200 degrees and turn it off.

- Leave your herbs on the stovetop, turning the stove on daily for about a week until the herbs are dry.

Teas are an attractive way to add fragrance and health benefits to soap. There are two methods of incorporating tea into soap: steeping and bleeding. To steep tea, the teabag is soaked in hot water for 2-5 minutes. This technique will lessen the amount of discoloration of your soap base when the tea is added. It is also used frequently when the herb or tealeaves are intended to add exfoliating properties. Not only can you add the solids, but you can also add a bit of the water, the tea was steeped in as well. Bleeding is the method that is chosen when the botanicals are being added for healing qualities or aromatherapy. In this method, the fresh or dried teas and herbs are attached directly to the heated soap base. This brings out the botanical's color, scent, and healing qualities.

If you want to include ingredients that will give the soap exfoliating powers consider adding:

- Coffee grounds
- Eucalyptus leaves
- Lavender buds
- Loofah
- Oatmeal
- Patchouli
- Poppy seeds
- Cornmeal
- Ground almonds

It may be beneficial to add vitamin E to the soap when using any dry additive. This will add moisture and decrease the amount of browning or oxidation that occurs. Capsules of vitamin E can be found with other vitamins at the pharmacy. Add 4-6 capsules per 4 ounces of soap.

Another way to stamp a bar of soap involves using a un-mounted rubber stamp. Follow this process:

- Take your stamp of choice and place it in your chosen mold with the textured design facing up.

- Melt 4 ounces of soap in the microwave. White or other light colors tend to work best.

- Add fragrance to the colored and melted soap if you desire.

- Use a small spray bottle to spritz the stamp with rubbing alcohol.

- Carefully pour the first layer of soap. An eyedropper can be used to get the soap without overflowing onto the stamp. With this first layer, you do not want to cover the top of the stamp.

- Allow this layer to harden for about five minutes.

- Prepare a second color of the soap. Make sure it is not too hot- shoot for less than 120 degrees.

- Spray the hardened soap with rubbing alcohol.

- Carefully pour the second layer, filling the mold.

- Allow the soap to harden for four hours at a minimum.

- Unmold the soap and peel back the rubber stamp.

- Any soap overhangs can be removed using a dental pick, paring knife, or anything else with an excellent point.

- Allow hardening entirely before storing

Layering is another easy way to create a fresh design. You can layer different colors, different textures (smooth, chunks, flakes, ribbons), or a combination of both. There are also some different designs you can add to your soaps using other soaps. If you grate up bits of various colored soaps, you can add them to a diverse base right before molding to achieve the look of confetti.

Chopping up pieces of soap will give a cobblestone effect. Another cool thing to do is use a vegetable peeler to make curls of soap. These curls can be embedded into a soap base.

Making soap balls is a great way to use up small amounts of leftover soap.

To do this:

- Grate up your leftover soap.

- If it has dried out, add a minimal amount of liquid to moisten the mix a bit. You can mix and match the colors in your soap balls, giving them a speckled or confetti look.

- Divide the grated soap and form it into oversized, loosely formed balls.

- Put one hand on top and one hand under the soap ball and squeeze down. Rotate the ball a little and squeeze again. Use gentle but steady pressure.

- Once they are the firmness, you want them, smooth the edges and allow them to cure for a week or two.

- These balls can be used on their own, or mini-balls can be added into another base for a fun decoration.

- It is also possible to make a checkerboard pattern within the soap. Follow this procedure:

- Make soap using your favorite technique.

- Mold into a square or rectangle and let harden. Do not let it cure; the fresher it is, the better this process will work.

- Use a knife to cut strips long enough to fit the length of the square mold you will be using.

- Once you are done cutting, lay 5 pieces (the number you need will depend on how big your mold is, but we will use specific numbers so you can get the idea) down with a space in between them.

- Start another layer putting two strips in the opposite direction.

- The next segment will go in the same direction as with the first 4 strips.

- Place 2 pieces the opposite way on the next layer.

- You will repeat this process to fill your mold with a grid pattern.

- Place the mold in a warm oven to meld the strips together just a little bit.

- Make a soap base using the cold process with a contrasting color, bringing it to a thin trace.

- Pour the lightly traced soap into the mold very carefully as not to disturb the grid pattern that you made.

- After pouring, gently tap the mold against your work surface to remove any air bubbles. The newly poured soap should have filled in the gaps in your grid pattern.

- Insulate as normal.

- After it hardens, remove from the mold and slice your soap in order to show off the design.

One unique soap design is felted soap. If you are familiar with knitting and wool, you have likely heard of felting. Felting soaps make for an individual looking bar that has excellent exfoliating properties from the wool. To felt soap, you will need several pieces of soap of varying shapes. This is a compelling way to use up batches of soap that you didn't find very pleasing to the eye. You will need 100% wool roving. In terms of equipment, you will need a towel, a washboard or sushi mat, old pantyhose, liquid soap, and a drying rack.

Follow these steps to create felted soap:

- Start by smoothing out the edges of your soap pieces.

- Pull off a section of the wool and wrap it around the soap in one direction.

- Choose another part of the wood and wrap it in the opposite direction.

- Place the covered soap in the foot-part of the pantyhose that have been cut off at the knee.

- Get the pantyhose wet by placing it under warm-hot running water.

- Squeeze some liquid soap over it to start the felting process.

- Rub the soap on the washboard or sushi mat, making sure to get all sides. This creates friction and allows the wool to felt.

- Keep rubbing the soap, stopping every once and a while to rinse it under water.

- After a few minutes, take the soap out of the stocking and see what you have.

- At this point, you could add more wool to make it thicker or combine different colors if it strikes your fancy.

- Put the soap back in the stocking and repeat the felting procedure until the wool is all matted down onto the soap.

- Remove the soap from the stocking.

- Rinse it in freshwater

- Blot dry with a towel.

- Place the soap on the drying rack and let it dry overnight. It will be ready to use the next day.

Chapter Four - Liquid Soap Making

The specialty of liquid soap making is likely probably the least demanding approach to make your soap at home. It's simple since dissolving down old bits of soap, or even a whole bar is brisk and basic. Liquid soap in its most straightforward structure is a bar soap that has had water added to it, until you don't have anything yet liquid left. The primary devices you will require are a pot, an estimating cup and a stove to warm everything.

You can likewise take it up an indent yet still keep it basic by adding a few scents to your soap or fundamental oils alongside a touch of shading. Generally, however, liquid soaps are typically placed into a compartment where you usea hand siphon, and usually, these are not regularly transparent, so shading doesn't need to be a thought

The main thing you accomplish for liquid soap making is to take a bar of soap, or even old pieces, and mesh them as finely as could reasonably be expected. At the point when they get too little, go through a blade to cut them, making a point to get it as fine as would be prudent. The subsequent stage is to place the ground soap into a cup with estimations as an afterthought and add water to approach the measure of ground soap.

The most challenging part of liquid soap making is the diluting process. If you use too little liquid, then you may see your soap start to form a skin, or it globs up in the bottle. If you add too much liquid, then you won't see a good lather.

It's important to make sure you follow your recipe to the letter, or you will run into problems. For the most part, liquid soap making is the easiest of all the soaps that you can make at home. Knowing this, you will probably be fine, and your recipe will work each time.

One of the most common reasons these days to use liquid soap is to help stop the spread of germs. The result, besides helping to prevent the spread of the flu germ, was a forty percent decrease in gastrointestinal problems.

Nowadays, it should be standard practice for every sink to have some liquid soap on the side for cleanliness as well as protection during flu seasons.

With liquid soap, you can add any number of essential oils that also serve as anti-bacterial agents. Oregano and tea tree oil are both high for this, but there are too many others to choose from. You can even blend them with other essential oils for an even more pleasant smell and yet still have a compelling product—one note of caution.

It is not advisable to use perfumed fragrances in combination with essential oils and still expect to have a compelling product. You also need to take into consideration that if guests are using liquid soap, and they have skin problems, then perfumed soap may not be to their liking. For guest bathrooms, it is suggested that you stick to all-natural ingredients whenever possible.

One thing that recently has become very popular is liquid face soap. My favorite is goat's milk. A simple recipe is to reduce your water content by about eight ounces, then add 0.2 ounces of potassium hydroxide for every twelve ounces of goat's milk. This will cause the goat's milk fat to saponify. It's that simple, and you will have a fantastic face soap that can easily be used daily.

The main thing to remember with liquid soap making is that it is the most straightforward technique around and probably the most foolproof. It's a great way to get started making soap or introducing your children to the beautiful world of soap making at home.

For what reason would you need to make a Liquid Soap?

Before making liquid soap, you have to wonder why you need to make liquid soap, does liquid soap have any edge over bar soaps? These are relevant inquiries that ought to be posed before diving into making any soap. I have a few hints regarding why you should include the creation of liquid soap to your item lineup.

- **Liquid soap has preferred edges over bar soap.**

Liquid soap is gainful, regardless of what you look like at it. In any event, considering the expense of liquid soap bundling (a jug and siphon), you can get more cash-flow selling liquid soap, then you can selling bar soap. Numerous customers consider liquid soap a better quality thing and will pay more for the comfort and look of liquid soap. Furthermore, the expense of products sold when making liquid soap is lower (a lot higher level of liquid soap is clean water contrasted with bar soap).

- **Twenty to thirty-year-olds favor liquid soap over bar soap.**

I have perused many articles that state youthful grown-ups favor liquid soap and body wash over bar soap. While I'm by and by an enthusiast of bar soap, when you are ready to go, you need to oblige what your real market needs. Regardless of whether your objective is more seasoned than recent college grads, in the long run, that may change over the long haul, or you may find that your objective market additionally appreciates the accommodation of liquid soap.

- **Liquid soap is the ideal item for a visitor washroom.**

There is a significant market for matched liquid soap and moisturizer sets for the visitor restroom and the kitchen. Indeed, even bar soap sweethearts like me comprehend that this set is a progressively costly answer for engaging.

Step by step instructions to make Natural Liquid Soap

Making your soap is moderately simple and requires ingredients you likely have, or can without much of a stretch get. Soap involves the utilization of potassium hydroxide, otherwise called lye, which can be dangerous to work with. For whatever length of time that you take as much time as necessary and fare thee well, you can securely make the liquid soap that you can use to top off all the soap distributors in your home.

There are a couple of strategies to make liquid soap, yet the most widely recognized approach is to create a soap glue using the hot procedure technique. The soap glue looks a great deal like warm procedure bar soap that has not yet solidified. The essential contrast between liquid soap and bar soaps is that potassium hydroxide (KOH) is used instead of sodium hydroxide (NaOH) for the lye arrangement.

There are some different contrasts between the two procedures, which I will cover further down. When you make the glue for liquid soap, you weaken the paste with water or another liquid. At that point, you can include any aroma or shading that you might want and presto! You have liquid soap!

Ingredients

Making Liquid Soap from a Bar

- 1 characteristic bar of soap of your decision
- 950 grams of water
- Essential oil of your decision (discretionary)

Pick a bar of natural soap. You can useany bar you like. The completed item will acquire its properties (like fragrance) from the bar you pick, so ensure that you choose one that you want. Making liquid soap from a bar of soap is a lot quicker and more secure than making soap without any preparation, as you won't need to work legitimately with any lye.

- Your completed item may be as "normal" as the bar of soap you pick. When explicitly attempting to make ordinary soap, ensure you have perused the ingredients list on the bar you are using.

Cut or mesh the soap into a skillet. The more finely you grind the soap, the simpler it will be to consolidate it with water.

- An ordinary kitchen grater will take care of business fine and dandy. If you use a grater that you use in your kitchen for nourishment, ensure that you flush it thoroughly before using it once more.

Include water. Use around 950 grams of water (approximately 4 cups) for a customarily measured bar of soap. You may modify the sum marginally, relying upon how thick you need the subsequent soap to be.

- Using considerably less water, about 350g, you can make a cream-like soap that can be used for shaving.

- You can differ the water sum contingent upon the exact thickness you need, using the above sums as a rule.

Carry the blend to a stew and mix until joined.

- The soap and water will take approximately 15 minutes to consolidate. At the point when it is done, it ought to have a foamy, soupy look.

- Before proceeding onward, let the blend cool for around 15 minutes. Rehash this whole advance if the blend is getting isolated.

Include essential oils. You can decide to skirt this progression if you would prefer not to add any extra aromas to your soap. If you would like to add essential oils to make your aroma, it is ideal, to begin with, an impartial, scentless soap.

- Essential oils are solid; a couple of drops is all you need. Permanently put a couple of drops into the blend and mix all together.

Let the soap sit for 24 hours. It takes about between a half and an entire day for the soap to completely "gel." You can leave the soap in a similar dish you used previously, or move it to another compartment.

- If you shake the soap and it holds its gel-like consistency, it is prepared to use.

- Make sure you include essential oils only after the soap has cooled and sat for 24 hours.

Empty the soap into gadgets. The soap will be prepared to useright away.

Making Liquid Soap from Scratch

When making a lot of soap that you probably won't useat the same time, ensure that you store the abundance in a perfect, fixed compartment.

- 100 grams of potassium hydroxide
- 170 grams of water
- 350 grams of olive oil
- 150 grams of coconut oil
- 850 grams of water (separate from the primary water)

Section 1: Preparing

- **Wear your protective apparel**. You are working with synthetic compounds that can cause harm to your skin. Make a point to keep your skin secured consistently. Defensive apparatus incorporates:

- Safety goggles/glasses. These are important to shield your eyes from any synthetic compounds that may sprinkle up.

- A long-sleeved shirt.

- Protective gloves.

- **Set up your kitchen scale**. Using a scale permits you to quantify your ingredients.

- Zero out the scale, making sure to put the empty vessel you will use on top.

- **Measure out the necessary ingredients**. Measure the water (170g or 850g), potassium hydroxide (100g), olive oil (350g) and coconut oil (150g) into independent dishes or holders, so they are fit to be joined with each progression.

- Ensure that you use a dry bowl or compartment for the potassium hydroxide. You don't need it to contact water until you are making the soap.

Section 2: Making the Soap

- **Mix the oils over low warmth.**

- Add 150 grams of coconut oil.

- Add 350 grams of olive oil to the coconut oil.

- Stir the oils together quickly; at that point, leave over low warmth while doing the subsequent stage.

- **Measure 100 grams of potassium hydroxide and 170 grams of water**. Use your kitchen scale and be mindful of quantifying precisely.

- 100 grams of potassium hydroxide

- 170 grams of water

- Set aside.

- **Empty the water into an empty bowl**. At that point, include the potassium hydroxide gradually and mix until the arrangement is clear. Cautioning: Do not pour the water over the potassium hydroxide! This can cause the concoction to respond and sprinkle up dangerously.

- Mix in a very much ventilated territory. If you are inside, open the windows.

- The mixture will warm up, so let it cool before proceeding onward.

- Combining water and potassium hydroxide will cause a compound response. This is ordinary, yet be cautious. Continuously make sure to keep your goggles on all through the procedure.

- **Add the water mixture to the oil mixture**.

- Pour gradually to stay away from sprinkles.

- Keep the zone very much ventilated.

- Ensure the whole mixture is filled the oil.

- **Mix by hand for five to ten minutes.**

- You need to guarantee that the oils, water, and potassium hydroxide are completely and mixed all together.

- **Mix with a submersion blender until the soap comes to "follow."** Immersion blenders are, in some cases, called "stick blenders." This will assist you in accomplishing the correct consistency in your soap a lot quicker than mixing totally by hand.

- Trace is a pudding-like consistency. If you can haul the blender out from the soap, and the round layout of the mixer remains marginally brought up in the soap for a couple of seconds, it has accomplished trace.

- If you don't have a submersion blender, you can mix by hand. Be that as it may, this will radically expand the measure of time the soap takes to accomplish follow.

- **Keep warming over low warmth for a few hours, blending each half-hour.** Coming back to mix is typically a significant piece of the procedure. Ensure the soap doesn't separate.

- The soap will be done when it takes after a reasonable jam.

- Nearly completed soap will be difficult, if certainly feasible, to mix.

- **Test the soap.** Include a modest quantity of soap to a limited quantity of bubbling water in the in 1:2 extent. You've made the base for your soap, yet it isn't correctly prepared to use.

- If, when mixed, the arrangement is clear, you're finished!

- If the mixture is a smooth white, at that point, return it to the warmth source and keep warming for an additional thirty minutes and rehash until the arrangement is clear.

Section 3: Finishing the Process

- **Heat the 850 grams of water to the point of boiling.** At that point, consolidate the water with the jam arrangement you have made.

- Stir until totally mixed and then remove the warmth and let the soap cool.

- **Give rest access to a container or other fixed compartment.** You should let your liquid soap rest for an all-inclusive timeframe. Soap may need to rest from a time of a day or two up to a few weeks.

- The soap will be prepared to use when it cools, however letting it sit will include clearness that you may want.

- **Empty the soap into containers**. You will probably have made more soap than will fit in one gadget, so disperse your liquid soap into containers for use around your home.

- When making a lot of soaps that you probably won't use at the same time, ensure that you store the overabundance in a perfect, fixed holder.

Tips for Making Liquid Soap and Precaution

Here is a portion of the things I've learned in the course of the most recent year of making liquid soap, so you won't need to learn them the most challenging way possible

If you need to upgrade your shower understanding - say farewell to strong soap and take a stab at making liquid soap. Making a liquid soap isn't as straightforward as making strong soap, although not even excessively confounded. Soap improvement begins with an essential concoction response among oils and soluble bases. The liquid soap is framed by the blend of fat (oil) and a solid arrangement of sodium and potassium hydroxide.

For strong soaps, sodium hydroxide is used, and different kinds of oils are used. However, to make it, for the most part, coconut oil is favored in a blend of delicate oils (like olive oil). The use of hard oil is additionally useful for liquid soap. Yet, if you need to clarify liquid one, at that point use of delicate oil is prescribed.

As you are concocting your liquid soap, try different things with different sorts of oils/fats (delicate or hard). Not every single delicate oil carries on incomparable example. Guarantee keeping up an appropriate parity of foam and saturating.

Elements For Making Liquid Soap:

For making liquid one, you will require these fixings in an equivalent amount:

- 7 oz. coconut oil
- oz. sunflower oil
- oz. KOH (Potassium Hydroxide)
- sublimated water for sodium and KOH mixture
- 40 oz. concentrated water to weaken the soap glue
- Boric corrosive
- 3 oz. scent or basic oils
- Colorant or soap color, as wanted.

Types of gear Needed For Making Liquid Soap

Liquid soap making requires different kinds of equipment and actualizes like a huge simmering pot, a thermometer, scale, estimating cups, potato mesher, stick blender, and so on.

Steps To Follow For Liquid Soap Making

- **Mix The Ingredients** - Mix all the oils in the equivalent amount in an enormous stewing pot on low fire. As the oils are warming up, mix sodium and potassium hydroxide in the water, observing the standard lye-production process. Exercise alert using burning potash, as it is somewhat unpredictable and, if not handled appropriately, can hurt. At the point when the lye-water is mixed, gradually include it into the hot oil mixture. Mix the mixture and later mix it using a stick blender.

- **Follow The Soap** - This procedure tests your understanding! Contingent on your mixture and amount, it might set aside an extended effort to find a good pace—30 minutes or more). Make a thick glue and guarantee no liquid is left before moving to the subsequent stage.

- **Cook The Paste** - Place the soap follow on warmth and give the mixture a decent mix, spread with the top, and pause. It might take approx—3-4 hours for this soap to cook. Continue blending the mixture after every 20-30 minutes. After the specified time, it will get rich for the most part Vaseline type.

- **Test The Mixture** - Add two ounces of water and one ounce ofc, mix it until the mixture disintegrates in water.

- **Weaken The Paste** - Bring the glue to bubble and continue blending with spoon or potato mesher for a couple of moments. Remove the warmth and spread the mixture with a cover. After the soap is disintegrated in water, kill it and include scent. Put the mixture on heat again at 180 degrees. In a different compartment include killing arrangement boric corrosive and boric arrangement. Pour the neutralizer in the soap mixture and mix well. Afterward, include scent or shading. Make the most of your liquid soap.

Tip: You can't super fat liquid soap to a similar degree that you can with bar soap.

The maximum you can superfat liquid soap is around 3%. In any case, a 3% superfat is, in reality, high if you need to include an aroma! I have taken in this exercise again and again because I made sure there must be an approach to make an 8% superfat liquid soap. Sadly, my clients like scented soaps, and when you include either essential oils or aroma oils to an exceptionally superfatted soap, it isolates. (And it looks exceptionally unappealing when that occurs.)

Tip: Some oils are more appropriate for making liquid soap than others.

The most widely recognized oils used in liquid soap making are olive oil, coconut oil and castor oil. I prescribe your first formula is one from Jackie's book using those three oils.

Coconut oil enables the liquid soap to glue saponify; in addition to it includes that foam support you know it for. Different oils that are high in immersed unsaturated fats like fat, cocoa spread, shea margarine and grease present difficulties (for the most part, darkness) in the liquid soap that you might need to handle not far off if you need to use them.

Olive oil helps keep the liquid soap thicker, while likewise being saturating, and castor oil does something unusual in liquid soap (only as it does in bar soap)!

Tip: Most liquid soaps are more slender than you may anticipate.

The more significant part of the liquid soaps we experience financially is surfactant-based items and not a natural soap. Olive oil-based liquid soaps will be thicker than coconut oil-based liquid soaps, so you'll need to remember that when using different plans.

If you choose to make a 100% coconut liquid soap for dishwashing or cleaning, it will be water-slim. If you need to thicken it, you should include a thickener or something to that effect. Including a thickener isn't the apocalypse. However, an exercise numerous individuals gain proficiency in the most challenging way possible!

Tip: Liquid soap making requires tolerance!

I am a hot procedure soap maker, so I am used to beginning and completing a cluster of soap FAST! Be that as it may, the weakening procedure in liquid soap works best when you give it time. Be set up for this and don't surge it!

It is more straightforward over the long haul to include a little water an opportunity to weaken than it is to manage a liquid soap that has an excessive amount of water added. So include your weakening water gradually, give it time, and show restraint.

Tip: Some added substances can cause issues when making liquid soap.

A well-known approach to make liquid soap thicker is to use a saline solution instead of the water in your lye arrangement. Like different added substances and changes in conventional liquid soap making, this technique has disadvantages. The most significant issue is that using saltwater in your lye arrangement can cloud the liquid soap. It likewise has the chance of hindering foam.

Tip: Making lye arrangement with KOH is unquestionably different than NaOH.

Potassium hydroxide (KOH) doesn't produce as a lot of warmth as sodium hydroxide (NaOH) does, so your lye water will cool all the more rapidly with KOH. You additionally need to make a point to mix when you add the KOH to the water to enable it to break down. Heads up: making a lye arrangement with KOH additionally makes a popping sound that astonished me the first run through!

Tip: Be cautious about weakening your soap glue with something besides pure water.

I am specifically alluding to what is designated "bug nourishment." Goat milk, muds and different botanicals in liquid soap can make a rearing ground for form and microbes. Regardless of whether you decide to include an additive, a portion of those added substances will test the restrictions of what an additive can do. Best to be as cautious as possible!

If you make a liquid soap with a low to no superfat and just weaken with filtered water, you ought not to require an additive. Make sure to use great assembling rehearses (GMP) to guarantee your items and compartments don't get defiled, however.

Tip: Liquid soap quite often should be tried and balanced.

Potassium hydroxide (KOH) isn't as unadulterated as sodium hydroxide (NaOH), and it separates all the more rapidly. Regardless of whether you are careful about estimating your fixings, you may end with a soap that is either lye substantial or superfatted. A cool aspect regarding liquid soap is that both of those issues are anything but difficult to fix after your liquid soap is weakened!

You can use two techniques to decide whether your liquid soap has overabundance oil or lye:

To check for abundance oil, mix a little piece of your thoroughly cooked glue with clean water. If it isn't smooth, at that point, your oils are saponified. Shady is alright, smooth isn't. If your soap has unsaponified oils, you can add some broke up KOH answer for saponifying the additional oils.

To test for abundance lye, you can use phenolphthalein drops in your weakened glue. Phenolphthalein drops check an answer for a little scope of pH, turning light pink to dim maroon if the arrangement has a pH somewhere in the range of 8 and 9.8.

If you add a drop of phenolphthalein to your liquid soap and it turns pink, you have abundance lye. Including broke up citrus extract is one strategy you can use to kill it, or using stearic corrosive is another. The two techniques and estimations for them are shrouded in detail in Jackie's book. If the weakened liquid soap doesn't turn pink when phenolphthalein drops are included, you are a great idea to go.

Tip: Test your aroma before adding it to your entire group of liquid soap.

The last advance before packaging your liquid soap is to include aroma (if wanted). Be set up for different scent oils and essential oils to respond with your liquid soap! It's always a smart thought to test your aroma in a little example of your liquid soap for, in any event, twenty-four hours. A few scents cause blurring, partition, thickening, or in any event, diminishing. I exceptionally recommend you test a limited quantity of completed liquid soap with your aroma before you add it to your whole group.

Safeguards:

Lye - a solid arrangement of sodium and potassium hydroxide can hurt your skin (may even consume), eyes (may cause visual deficiency), or open body parts because of its hazardous nature. Wear gloves and wear goggles when handling potassium hydroxide. Store it in a water/air proof container away from the compass of kids and pets. Burning potash causes skin tingling. After utilization, wash your hands with vinegar and clean water.

Liquid Soap Recipes

Proceeding onward to the business end of things, we will be taking a gander at 25 different recipes for natively constructed liquid soap-related items. To begin things off, here are five recipes for a regular soap you can attempt at home.

- Shampoos

You may be pondering that since you can without much of a stretch purchase your soap at the closest comfort store, for what reason should you experience the bother of making your soap at home? The truth is that there are various advantages to making your soap.

We should specify some of them:

- Making soap at home is simpler than you might suspect. As you will find in the recipes recorded underneath, you don't need to do much except joining the ingredients and shaking them well. In this way, you don't need to place in as well much exertion.

- The expense of natively constructed soap is significantly lower than what you would pay for a jug of soap from a good brand. This way, you can set aside money.

- You can modify the ingredients and their arrangement dependent on your specific needs. If you have a dry scalp, you can make a soap that treats that particular issue. This extravagance of customization isn't accessible to you if you purchase business soap.

- You can guarantee that the soap you make is regular and without any handled or refined ingredients. Some business brands of soap guarantee to deliver an essential item; however, they use some engineered materials to get the correct thickness, shading and scent.

- In particular, you can keep away from the poisons and destructive components that are mainly part of business soaps. The toxins can harm your hair instead of assisting it with holding its appearance.

As should be obvious, there are various advantages of making your soap. Things being what they are, how might you approach doing that? Here are five extraordinary recipes for making soap at home

Basic

The recipe for a basic natively constructed soap is imperative to learn. Almost all other recipes for soap follow a similar base.

Ingredients:

- ½ cup liquid Castile Soap (Buy any variation you need)

- 1 cup of refined water

- ½ teaspoon Avocado Oil (Substitute with Jojoba or Grape seed Oil if you need)

Directions:

- Take a little bowl and pour in all ingredients.

- Stir the mixture till the ingredients consolidate well.

- Empty the mixture into a jug or plastic compartment.

- Shake a long time before you need to use the soap.

As guaranteed, the recipe for a basic natively constructed soap is very straightforward and uncomplicated. Presently it's an ideal opportunity to go over some different recipes.

Herbal

The herbal soap is extraordinary for your hair wellbeing and can be used by individuals with all kinds of hair.

Ingredients:

- Two tablespoons Tea Tree Oil

- 1 cup refined Water

- Three tablespoons dried Rosemary

- ½ teaspoon Avocado Oil

- ¼ cup liquid Castile Soap

- One tablespoon Lemongrass

Guidelines:

1. Empty the filtered water into a pan and put over medium-high warmth. Heat to the point of boiling.

2. Add herbs to the boiled water and leave it to soak for around 40 minutes—Channel the water, evacuating any rosemary or lemongrass fantasies.

3. Move the liquid to a compartment, ideally a glass holder. Include the oils and Castile soap to the liquid. Stir well until the oil, soap and water are mixed all together. This may take in excess of a few minutes.

4. Allow the mixture to cool and then empty into a container with a froth siphon. Use the soap at whatever point you need.

Sweet

In what manner can soap be sweet? Here, we aren't discussing the flavor of the soap, yet rather its smell.

Ingredients:

- ¼ teaspoon Avocado Oil
- 8 drops Coconut Fragrance Oil
- 1 cup refined Water
- 8 drops Vanilla Fragrance Oil
- ¼ cup liquid Castile Soap

Directions:

- In a mixing bowl, consolidate all the ingredients.
- Stir the mixture to guarantee the ingredients mix well.
- Check the aroma to judge whether the mixture is excellent.
- Move the substance to a jug.

Anybody and everybody can use the sweet soap. If you need your hair to smell decent, this is the ideal recipe for you.

Apple Cider Vinegar Rinse

If you are attempting to dispose of dandruff and grime from your hair, using Apple Juice Vinegar Rinse likely could be an incredible alternative. Not exclusively does it helps keep your hair clean; however, it likewise reestablishes its imperativeness and dynamic quality.

Ingredients:

- 1 cup Distilled Water
- 1/3 cup of crude Apple Cider Vinegar

Directions:

- Consolidate the water and vinegar in a jug or plastic holder.
- Shake well, so the ingredients mix flawlessly together.

For using Apple Cider Vinegar Rinse, you need to cleanser your hair first. You can use any of the three choices recorded previously. Wash your hair thoroughly to guarantee there is no cleanser buildup left. Delicately focus on the vinegar flush into your scalp. Ensure you spread every single piece of your head. At that point, let the hair sit for a few minutes before flushing off the vinegar wash.

Use cold water to get the best outcomes. The main catch is that your hair will smell like apple juice vinegar, yet that can be managed by applying conditioner to your hair a while later or in any event, shampooing it once more.

Luster

Who doesn't need their hair to seem gleaming and hold its unique radiance? However, after some time, your hair will lose its sheen and appearance because of dryness and different components. Making and applying a radiance cleanser to your hair regularly will assist you with reestablishing the sparkle you are searching for.

Ingredients:

- ¼ teaspoon Lemon Essential Oil
- ¼ cup Castile Soap
- 2 tablespoons Sweet Almond Oil
- 1 cup Distilled Water
- 2 tablespoons dried Rosemary

Directions:

- Add Rosemary to the clean water and heat to the point of boiling. Let the mixture soak for 40 minutes. Strain the leaves.
- Include the rest of the ingredients to the mixture. Stir well, so they mix appropriately.
- Move the substance to a jug or plastic holder.

Store the luster cleanser in a cool spot.

- Shower Gels

Causing your shampoos at home to can do ponders for the appearance and soundness of your hair and scalp. Things being what they are, shouldn't something be said about the remainder of your body? For that, you can make shower gels at home and use them for taking long, loosening up showers. Like shampoos, business shower gels likewise contain a few materials that are hurtful for your skin.

You can evade the issues a great many people face by following the recipes given right now, making shower gels at home.

Interestingly, there are a few aromas you can decide on.

Here are five of the best:

Basic

To begin with, making shower gel at home, here is an essential recipe you can attempt first.

Ingredients:

- 1 standard Soap Bar
- 1 cup of Distilled Water

Guidelines:

- Cut or mesh the soap bar into little pieces or drops. The pieces ought to be small enough that they get broke up no problem at all.
- Empty the filtered water into a pot and toss in the soap bar drops.
- Heat the water to the point of boiling and keep on stewing till the soap softens totally.
- Stir the water till the soap and water structure a smooth gel-like mixture.
- Move to a mixing bowl and let cool.
- Empty the mixture into a container and use it when vital.

Pear

The essential recipe for making shower gel stays the equivalent. The primary difference is in the aroma. Here is the recipe for pear shower gel.

Ingredients:

- 1 cup of Distilled Water
- 1 tablespoon of Glycerin
- 1 bar of unscented Glycerin Soap
- ½ cup of Pear Juice
- 3 drops of Lemon Essential Oil
- 5 drops of Pear Fragrance Oil

Directions:

The procedure continues as before as that for making essential shower gel. The difference is that you need to mix the oils, juice and glycerin into the mixture when it is ready.

You can likewise substitute pear with apple if you favor the smell of apples over pears.

Strawberry and Lemon

This is a fascinating mix you will unquestionably not find in any financially accessible shower gel: Strawberry and Lemon.

Ingredients:

- 3 enormous solidified Strawberries
- 1 tablespoon of Aloe Vera Gel

- ½ tablespoon of unscented, regular Liquid Soap
- 1 teaspoon of salt
- 5 drops of Strawberry Fragrance Oil
- 8 drops of Lemon Essential Oil

Guidelines:

- Defrost the solidified strawberries till they mellow. Hurl into a blender and puree till smooth.
- Move the pureed strawberries into a bowl and join with salt.
- Add the rest of the ingredients to the bowl and mix well.

You should use the shower gel immediately.

Orange

This one is a different recipe as it doesn't expect you to use soap.

Ingredients:

- 1 teaspoon of Cane Sugar
- 1 cup of Distilled Water
- 8 drops of Essential Lemon Oil
- 2 tablespoons of Glycerin
- 2 drops of Orange Food Coloring
- 1 tablespoon of Jojoba Oil
- 4 tablespoons of Aloe Vera Gel

- 1 teaspoon of Arrowroot

Directions:

- Consolidate all the ingredients in a bowl and mix well together until they are smooth.
- Include the nourishment shading and stir well.
- Move the gel into a press container and use inside a day.

You can use grapefruit, lemon or lime instead of orange.

Vanilla Rose

Vanilla rose shower gel is shockingly simple to make.

Ingredients:

- 1 unscented regular Soap Bar
- 1 cup Distilled Water
- 10 drops Vanilla Extract
- 8 drops Rose Essential Oil

Guidelines:

- Adhere to the instructions for essential shower gel.
- Add the concentrate and oil to the gel and mix well.

Your vanilla rose shower gel is prepared!

Laundry Soaps

Having secured shampoos and shower gels, presently, it is time we proceed onward to cleansers. A great many people probably won't know about the way that the methods used for making liquid clothing soaps are very like the ones followed to make hand soaps and shampoos. In this way, while you are finding out about them, why not give clothing cleanser a go?

Front-Load/Top-Load Machines

Here is a recipe for clothing soap that works impeccably in front-burden and top-load machines.

Ingredients:

- 4 cups of hot Distilled Water
- ½ cup of Borax
- 1 Detergent Bar, grind!.
- 1 cup of Washing Soda

Guidelines:

- Join the soap and water in a pan and boil till the soap is disintegrated.
- Fill a container of water and pour in all ingredients, including the soap mixture.

Stir and spread the can and leave medium-term with the goal that the mixture thickens.

- Move the mixture to a soap container for simple use.

Basic/Essential

The recipe for essential clothing soap is straightforward to follow.

Ingredients:

- 1 Detergent Bar, grind!.
- ½ cup Vinegar
- 4 cups Distilled Water

Directions:

- Put the ground soap into a pot and pour the water in. Heat to the point of boiling and add the vinegar.
- Let the mixture stand till it chills off and move to soap siphons.

Berries

If you love berries and need your garments to possess a scent like berries, you can attempt the recipe for Berry liquid cleanser.

Ingredients:

- ½ cup of Vinegar
- 1 cup of Berries (of your decision)
- 4 cups of Distilled Water

Guidelines:

- Join the ingredients in a pan and bring to a low boil. Spot the cover on and stew for around 30 minutes. Continue stirring the mixture so that the berries break into little pieces.

- Expel the cover and stew for a further 30 minutes at low warmth.
- Strain into a bowl and let cool.

Orange

The orange aroma is very refreshing, which is one motivation behind why it is so well known.

Ingredients:

- 1 cup of cut Oranges
- 4 cups of Distilled Water
- ½ cup of Vinegar

Directions:

- Consolidate the ingredients in a pot and bring to a low boil. Spot the cover on and stew for around 30 minutes. Continue stirring the mixture so that the natural product breaks into little pieces.
- Expel the top and stew for a further 30 minutes at low warmth.
- Strain into a bowl and let cool.

Lemon

Ingredients:

- 1 cup of cut Lemons
- ½ cup of Vinegar
- 4 cups of Distilled Water

Guidelines:

- Join the ingredients in a pot and bring to a low boil. Spot the cover on and stew for around 30 minutes. Continue stirring the mixture so that the lemons break into little pieces.

- Evacuate the cover and simmer for a further 30 minutes at low warmth.

- Strain into a bowl and let cool.

Hand Soaps

Hand soaps are an essential piece of the month to month shopping list. You may not be ready to understand not having hand soap at home. Most households spend a reasonable measure of cash on purchasing hand soaps each month. Hence, if you figure out how to make your own, you can set aside a ton of money. There is no shortage of recipes as far as hand soaps are concerned.

Fundamental

The fundamental technique is the thing that you need to follow for the rest of the recipes also.

Ingredients:

- 1 bar of soap, ground
- 1 cup of Distilled Water
- ½ teaspoon of Essential Oil
- 1 tablespoon of Glycerin

Directions:

- Consolidate the ingredients in a pot and put on medium warmth.

- Heat the mixture to the point of boiling and let stew till the soap breaks up totally.

- Move the substance to a soap siphon and use it.

All-Natural

Every ordinary soap is incredible for your skin, notwithstanding being environmentally friendly.

Ingredients:

- 1 cup of Distilled Water
- 1 tablespoon of Glycerin
- 1 bar of unscented Baby Mild Liquid Soap
- ½ teaspoon of Grapefruit Essential Oil

Directions:

- Mix the ingredients. The perfect proportion is 1 cup of water and ¼ teaspoon essential oils for each 1 oz of soap. You need to modify it in like manner.

- Stir till the mixture is smooth and move to compartments.

Coconut

Did you realize that coconut oil is an ideal substitute for Glycerin? This allows you to make coconut hand liquid Soap!

Ingredients:

- 1 tablespoon of Coconut Oil
- 1 gallon of Distilled Water

- 1 bar soap

Guidelines:

- Mesh the soap into a pan.
- Into the pan, pour water and include oil.
- Put over medium-high heat cook until the soap disintegrates totally.

Ensure that the mixture doesn't boil.

Pigeon

Pigeon is one of the most famous soap brands. You can make your Dove hand liquid soap at home!

Ingredients:

- 1 gallon of Distilled Water
- 1 bar Dove Soap
- 1 tablespoon of Glycerin
- ½ tablespoon of Grapefruit Essential Oil

Directions:

You need to follow a similar strategy as that for fundamental hand liquid soap without any changes.

Infant

The skin of little youngsters expects you to be cautious about the sort of soap you use.

Ingredients:

- 1 bar Baby Soap (any brand)
- 1 gallon of Distilled Water
- 1 tablespoon of Glycerin

Directions:

Apply the method for making fundamental hand liquid soap. The only difference is that you don't need to use essential oils right now.

Salicylate-Free

A few people are hypersensitive to Salicylate. Since every business brand of soap has Salicylate, it is significant that you discover one that doesn't. You can make Sans Salicylate hand liquid soap at home.

Ingredients:

- 2 cups of hot Distilled Water
- 1 bar soap (ideally Olay or Dove)

Guidelines:

- Join the ingredients in a pot. Warmth till the soap breaks up in the water.
- Let it stand for 24 hours, stirring each hour or so till the mixture cools down.
- If you don't see the ideal smoothness, you can include one tablespoon of Glycerin.

Ivory

If you like ivory soap, you will appreciate making ivory liquid hand soap.

Ingredients:

- 1 bar Ivory Soap, grind!
- 12 cups of Distilled water

Guidelines:

- Put 4 cups of water and the soap into an enormous pot and boil until soap breaks down.
- Whisk the mixture till the soap mixes thoroughly.
- Include the rest of the cups of water and let it cool before using it.

Lavender

Lavender is one of the most famous aromas. You can get the stunning fragrance in your hand soap also.

Ingredients:

- 1 bar unscented soap, grind!
- 1 cup of Distilled Water
- 1 tablespoon of Glycerin
- 12 drops of Lavender Essential Oil

Guidelines:

The recipe continues as before. You may need to differ the quantity of drops of essential oil you put in relying upon the aroma that radiates.

Pomegranate - Rose

Pomegranate and rose likely could be a surprising blend; however, you will like it.

Ingredients:

- 2 bars of Pomegranate and Rose Soap
- 1 gallon of Water
- 2 tablespoons of Glycerin

Directions:

- Mesh the bars of soap into little pieces.
- Consolidate all ingredients, with ground soap, in a large pan or pot. Make sure the compartment is large enough for 1 gallon of water.
- Turn the stove on medium and warmth the mixture until the soap breaks down totally.
- Let the soap sit for about 12 hours.
- Move to holders and use them as hand soap.

Chocolate

Here is a recipe to end things on a high: chocolate hand soap!

Ingredients:

- 1 bar Chocolate Soap
- 1 cup of Distilled Water

- 1 tablespoon of Glycerin

Guidelines:

Follow the basic recipe precisely, and you can make yourself extraordinary smelling chocolate liquid hand soap!

Liquid Castile Soap

Ingredients:

- 24 ounces Olive Oil
- 16 ounces Coconut Oil
- ounces Potassium Hydroxide Lye Flakes
- 32 ounces Distilled Water
- 10 to 12 cups Distilled water

Directions:

- Include the Olive Oil and Coconut Oil to a substantial slow cooker and turn on high.
- While the oils are dissolving, place your 32 ounces of Distilled Water into a medium tempered steel bowl.
- Cautiously add the lye to the water and stir to break up.
- When the oils are warm and dissolved, cautiously include the lye arrangement into the slow cooker.

- Mix the oils and lye with a drenching blender. Mix quickly for five minutes or until the mixture starts to thicken. Cook for the following 30 minutes while mixing like clockwork.

- When the soap is too thick to even think about blending, place the top on the stewing pot and leave to cook on high for three hours.

- Return at regular intervals to the crease and stir the soap with a spatula or wooden spoon.

- After three hours, test the soap. Measure out an ounce of soap and include 4 ounces of boiling or high temp water. Stir tenderly until the soap is broken down. Permit it to cool; if it is dark or if oils buoy to the surface at that point, keep cooking for one more hour and retest. Something else, if it is clear, at that point, you can continue.

- Include 10 cups of filtered water to the simmering pot. Separate the soap as best as could reasonably be expected.

- Spot the top on the stewing pot and go to warm for 8 hours to medium-term and stir when you can.

- After 8 hours, if you notice lumps of soap or a tough skin framing, at that point, you should add another cup to two of filtered water.

- When the soap is completely disintegrated without any lumps, at that point, you can scoop your soap into wanted compartments.

Liquid Dish Soap

Ingredients:

- 1 ½ cups Boiling water
- ¼ cup Grated Bar Soap
- ¼ cup Liquid Castile Soap
- 2 ¼ teaspoon - 1 tablespoon Super Washing Soda
- ½ teaspoon Glycerin
- 15-40 drops Essential Oil Fragrance of your decision.

Directions:

- Boil water on the stove over medium/high warmth. Include the ground bar soap and stir until broken up.
- Expel from warm and fill the ideal compartment.
- Include the liquid castile soap, 2 ¼ teaspoons super washing pop and Glycerin. Stir completely.
- Permit the soap to sit medium-term with occasional stirring. If you need it thicker, at that point, warm it up and break down in another ¾ teaspoon washing pop and permit it to sit medium-term once more.
- If the soap is clumpy, place it in the blender or mix with a submersion blender.

- After you get the correct consistency, at that point, you can mix in wanted essential oils.

- Spot in a disperser holder of your decision, and you're all set.

Moisturizing Cream Hand Soap

Ingredients:

- 0.26 ounce Castor Oil
- 0.07 ounce Jojoba Oil
- 0.35 ounce Olive Oil
- 0.17 ounce Shea Butter
- 1-ounce Coconut Oil
- 0.7 ounce Palm Oil
- ounces Stearic Acid
- 1.8 ounces Glycerin
- 0.17-ounce Sodium Hydroxide Lye
- 0.89-ounce Potassium Hydroxide Lye
- ounces Distilled Water
- 0.08-ounce Melted Stearic Acid
- 0.13-ounce Glycerin mixed with the Stearic Acid
- ounces Aloe Juice or Water

- 0.88 ounce Aloe Juice
- 0.16-ounce Allantoin
- 0.08-ounce Kaolin Clay
- 0.16-ounce Hydrolyzed Silk
- 0.16 ounce Goat's Milk Powder

Directions:

- Preheat the grill to 250 degrees Fahrenheit.
- Spot oils/spread and first glycerin measure in a soap pot and warmth until merely liquefied.
- Add the two lyes to the water measure and put aside to cool.
- Add the lye water to the oils/margarine/glycerin mix and stick mix until smooth and uniform.
- Permit the soap to rest for a couple of moments.
- Spread the pot and spot in the stove for 45 minutes to 60 minutes.
- Check at regular intervals and stir.
- Warmth the stearic corrosive and Glycerin mix until liquefied and add to the hot soap.
- Mood killer the stove and leave the pot secured medium-term.
- Whip the soap until it disengages.

- Use a stick blender and switch back and forth between including the aloe juice and mixing until you accomplish the consistency of icing.

- Include added substances and stir by hand.

- Move to a glass or clay dish with a cover. Spread and solution for the least of about fourteen days.

- Test the surface and whip the soap. If it is too figure, you can include extra aloe juice ¼ teaspoon at once.

- Include shading and fragrance as wanted.

- Fill the ideal distributor.

Liquid Body Wash

Ingredients:

- 8 ounces of your favored bar soap
- 2 tablespoons Glycerin
- 1 gallon of water

Directions:

- Mesh the bar soap and spot in a stockpot with the water and Glycerin.

- Warmth on medium warmth until the soap is broken down.

- Remove from the heat and permit to cool for 10-12 hours.

- Beat with a hand mixer and add water varying to get the ideal consistency.
- Include any aroma you want.
- Channel into your ideal holder.

Foaming Liquid Soap

Ingredients:

- 245 ml Liquid Castile Soap Base
- 5 ml Vitamin E
- 10 drops Eucalyptus Lemon Essential Oil
- 10 drops Lavender
- Essential Oil

Directions:

- To use in a customary siphon or flip-top jug join ingredients, seal and foment to join.
- To use in an airless foamer, join the ingredients and then weaken with water in a 1:3-6 proportion until you have a flimsy and watery liquid. Upset to mix thoroughly. Immerse your jug and seal.

Charcoal Facial Cleanser

Ingredients:

- 0.5 ounce Cocoa Butter

- 0.25 ounce Shea Butter
- 3.5 ounces Liquid Castile Soap
- 1 teaspoon Liquid Soy Lecithin
- 2 ml Rosehip Seed Oil
- 15 drops Birch Tar Essential Oil
- 15 drops Rose Outright Blend
- 5 drops Vitamin E
- 5 drops Rosemary Extract
- 1 teaspoon Activated Charcoal Powder

Directions:

- Soften the Cocoa Butter and Shea Butters in a double boiler.
- Stir the Soy Lecithin into the dissolved spread until altogether consolidated.
- Tenderly stir in the Castile Soap.
- Stir in the Rosehip Seed Oil.
- Stir in the essential oils, Vitamin E and Rosemary Extract.
- Rush in the Activated Charcoal Powder.

- Fill a glass bottle with a cream siphon and permit to cool before utilizing it.

Honey and Dandelion Floral Liquid Soap

Ingredients:

- 8 ounces Coconut Oil
- 4 ounces Olive Oil infused with Dandelion
- 4 ounces Sunflower Oil
- 4 ounces Castor Oil
- 4.63 ounces Potassium Hydroxide Lye
- 13.75 ounces Dandelion Tea or Distilled Water
- 1 teaspoon nectar mixed with 1 teaspoon warm water
- Vegetable Glycerin
- Distilled Water

Directions:

- The initial step is to set up your Dandelion Tea. Spot 1 cup of Dandelion Blossoms in a heatproof shake and pour 1.5 cups of hot refined water over them. Permit the tea to infuse for 20 to 30 minutes at that point strain. Cool totally before utilizing in the soap recipe.
- Spot the cooled tea in hardened steel or heatproof holder. Include more filtered water if required.

- Add the lye to the dandelion tea and stir well. Put the lye arrangement in a safe spot.

- In a moderate cooker, join the oils and turn the warmth on low. Include the dandelion tea and lye arrangement. Hand stir for around 5 minutes until well mixed.

- Begin mixing with a stick blender until you accomplish follow.

- Stir in nectar and water mixture.

- Spread the moderate cooker and keep on low warmth. Check the soap every 30 minutes or somewhere in the vicinity and stirring each time.

- Keep cooking around 2 hours until you have a Vaseline consistency.

- Gauge your soap glue and duplicate the weight by 0.20 to get the measure of Glycerin required; at that point, double the pressure by 0.80 to understand how much Distilled Water you need.

- Join the Glycerin and water in a deep pan and heat to the point of boiling. Scratch the soap glue into the mixture at that point spread the skillet and mood killer the warmth, leaving the pot on the burner.

- Permit the mixture to come to room temperature, stirring and squashing at times.

- Heat the mixture back to the point of boiling more than once and permit to cool once more, stirring to separate massive protuberances.

- Keep the soap in a secured tempered steel prospect not many days, infrequently stirring until the entirety of the soap glue is broken up.

- Fill containers and permit to make do with a couple of more days.

Lavender and Oatmeal Body Wash

Ingredients:

- 3 cups Distilled water
- ¼ cup Oatmeal
- ¼ cup Liquid Castile Soap
- 6-12 drops Lavender Essential Oil
- 1 teaspoon Vitamin E Oil
- 2 teaspoon Jojoba or Avocado Oil

Directions:

- Heat the water to the point of boiling. Pour the boiling water over the cereal in a glass bowl. Permit to sit for one to two hours and then strain to evacuate the oats from the water. Dispose of the oats and put the water in a safe spot.

- Mix the castile soap, essential oil, Vitamin E and jojoba/avocado oil in a little bowl with speed until totally mixed.

- Pour enough of the soap/oil mixture to fill 10-15% of a frothing soap container.

- Empty the oats water into the container until practically full, and you're all set.

Moisturizing Soap

Ingredients:

- 1 cup of Liquid Castile Soap in the prefered fragrance
- 1 cup Refined Water
- 3 tablespoons Coconut Oil

Directions:

- Empty the liquid soap into a glass bowl and then include the water.
- Include the coconut oil and mix everything by stirring.
- Move to a container to use.

Liquid Laundry Soap

Ingredients:

- 1 cup exceptionally boiling water
- 1 cup castile soap, the aroma of your decision

- ½ cup washing soft drink

- ½ cup borax

Directions:

- Spot the borax and washing soft drink in a little pitcher.

- Include the high temp water and stir until completely broken up.

- Fill the ideal compartment and include castile soap.

- Top compartment and tilt to and fro to mix.

- Include cold water until the holder is full, leaving space to mix.

- Top the compartment again and tilt to and fro to mix.

- Permit cooling, infrequently shaking to mix.

Acing Your Liquid Soap Making

There are loads of valid justifications as to why you should ace liquid soap making, the most significant explanation being that you can tailor-make the soap for your skin type and aroma of your decision. Additionally, liquid soap making can be an extraordinary method for making thoughtful, customized gifts if you have a restricted spending plan.

Liquid soap making is finished by utilizing glycerin, which can be purchased from in mass from most drug stores or wellbeing nourishment stores. Glycerin is a thick, practically coagulated liquid that is delivered from creature fats. It is frequently added to excellence items and beauty care products because of its saturating properties. The bizarre thing about glycerin, in any case, is that in its unadulterated structure, it can really expel dampness from delicate skin and even cause rankling. Accordingly, it is always reasonable to wear elastic gloves when working with glycerin.

You can make an essential liquid soap that uses bar-soap as a base. Yet, I like to begin my liquid soap making without any preparation, utilizing the accompanying essential recipe, which I customize by using a few different varieties.

You will require:

- 6 ounces of water
- 3 ounces of potassium hydroxide
- 8 ounces of non-hydrogenated soybean oil
- 4 ounces of coconut oil
- 4 ounces of sunflower oil
- A large portion of a cup of glycerin
- Essential oil or a mix of oils of your decision

First, mix the water with the potassium hydroxide and leave it on one side. At that point, consolidate the oils together (not the essential oil) and warmth gradually, stirring admirably.

After the oils are very much mixed, carry the mixture to around 150 degrees F and stir in the water/potassium hydroxide mixture. Mix energetically to keep the different components from isolating. When the oils have quit ascending to the surface, permit the mixture to cool. You, at that point, let this mixture sit for a week or something like that, infrequently stirring to keep the oils from isolating.

At long last, include a large portion of a cup of glycerin and the measure of essential oil that invigorates the smell that you are focusing on, and then give the mixture a last stir. You would then be able to include water until the combination is the consistency you require - for a liquid soap include more water and for a body wash, include less. Fill siphon bottles, prepared for use.

Varieties - For a homegrown soap supplant, the 6 ounces of water with a mix of solid natural tea. Chamomile and mint function admirably as greens tea. Likewise, if you need all the more a body scour impact at that point, take a stab at including a touch of cereal into the mix, which will go about as a delicate exfoliator. You could likewise add nourishment colorings and even body sparkles for different outcomes. For more varieties, substitute the coconut and sunflower oil with various transporters, for example, almond oil or avocado and have a go at including different and fascinating mixes of oils.

Play around with your liquid soap making and recall as far as possible is your creative mind!

The most effective method to make Liquid Soaps for Babies.

Kids, particularly coddle, are valuable to us, and we wouldn't have any desire to use a brutal concoction made soap on them. If you have been making a natively constructed soap and you don't use a mixture loaded soap to yourself, for what reason would it be a good idea for you to use it for your infant? I have investigated different details to think of the conceivable wager creation for your baby's use.

What are the fundamental strides to take to make a substance-free liquid soap for kids?

The primary thing that I looked into is what are the ingredients that are the most perfect and mildest most appropriate for an infant. The essential oil is one of my interests since, dependent on my experience; its smell can be somewhat overpowering on occasion. Chamomile essential oil is the most reasonable for the infant because of its gentle aroma.

I likewise needed to discover what are the different ingredients that I can mix with my liquid soap? The use of synthetic concoctions, for example, potassium hydroxide can cause a bothering to infants, and so I needed to look at what is the other option. Ideally, I gained from an individual soap producer that in making liquid soap, you can abstain from utilizing lye or potassium hydroxide. It may not keep going extremely long, yet at any rate, you are guaranteed of a synthetic-free recipe.

Here are the essential strides to take to make your liquid soap for babies.

- Get a bar soap.

- Grate the bar soap utilizing my cheddar grater and put it in a safe spot.

- Boil some water and pour this onto the ground bar soap.

- Use proportion 2:1, which means for every 2 cups of liquid, mix one cup of the ground bar soap for each bunch. You may not make a ton since its average period of usability is shorter than the economically made liquid soaps since you are not utilizing any additives.

- Mix it utilizing a blender to ensure that your liquid soap will be smooth for your infant's touchy skin.

- Put a couple of drops of chamomile and lavender oil for mitigating impact, and then remix it well overall.

- t it cool for a few hours.

- Get a hand soap gadget for keeping your infant's liquid soap.

Step by step instructions to make liquid soap is so natural and fun as well. All in all, would you say you are presently persuaded that creating your own infant's liquid soap is the superb gift you can give your infant? Give it a shot, and I am sure that you will likewise appreciate a similar liquid soap for your very own use.

Chapter Five - Disinfecting Wipes

Hand sanitizers and disinfecting wipes have extraordinary pertinence in the present exceptionally contaminated condition. They work as defensive covers to shield against harmful organisms, which cause ailment. The regular use of these cleaning arrangements is the perfect method to keep up legitimate individual cleanliness and sanitation. Because of the rising demand for them, the market is stacked with a broad assortment of these items.

Consistently, large numbers of germs are spread around by our hands. These germs can be genuinely innocuous, and those with solid insusceptible frameworks will regularly oppose these germs effectively, yet they can be the cause of colds and belly bugs. Even though these are just minor sicknesses, germs can likewise be the cause of progressively genuine difficulties. They can also spread contamination in minor injuries, which brings about the increasingly authentic ailment. The spreading of these germs can be reduced substantially by keeping your hands perfect and observing fundamental guidelines of cleanliness.

A significant number of the germs on your hands can be executed by routinely washing your hands with soap and water. However, perhaps the most secure approach to eliminate germs is to use a hand sanitizer. Hand sanitizers contain alcohol and are extraordinarily figured to demolish up to 99.9% of germs and microbes. They were initially used in places where it is essential to keep up an elevated level of cleanliness; for example, emergency clinics, however, have gotten progressively well known for regular use.

You can make hand sanitizers as self-retaining gels that you apply as you would a hand cream. They ingest into your skin and clean your hands simultaneously. They are accommodating as you can keep a little container of sanitizer gel in your handbag or stash and apply it at whatever point you feel the need. These are so useful when a dreadful bug is going near. You can likewise make hand sanitizers as soap and disinfecting wipes.

It is likewise imperative to keep some fundamental cleanliness governs, particularly when you are getting ready or putting away nourishment. You ought to consistently wash your hands thoroughly before contacting nourishment and ensure that your work surface and utensils are, for the most part, perfect. Crude nourishments, particularly meat, ought to be put away at the correct temperature, and it is significant not to let crude meat come into contact with different nourishments. Defilement adds to the spreading of germs and contaminations, so to be sheltered, you should use separate sheets for cutting and getting ready meats, dairy items, wheat items and products of the soil. These are only a couple of the cleanliness rules for nourishment planning.

Essentially, we are continually getting germs and microscopic organisms on our hands. These germs can spread and cause sickness and disease; however, by keeping your hands clean, utilizing a hand sanitizer, and by remembering cleanliness consistently, you can significantly lessen the spreading of contamination.

At the point when you have to clean your hands and don't approach the sink and bar of soap, you can necessarily venture into your pocket or tote for hand wipes. Nothing gives such a snappy cleanup as these individual moist disposable clothes. They are intended for comfort and accessibility. Regardless of whether for your hands or your child's, you will be so happy, you had one in your pocket.

Cleaning Your Toddler's Hands

You won't need to stress over the stuff your little child contacts - and they contact everything! When you see that the individual is going after things that are not precisely alluring, you can pull out the hand wipes and clean their fingers from whatever mess they have gotten themselves into.

Remember Your Hands

They're extraordinary for grown-ups as well. How often do you end up with something on your hands and wishing you had an approach to clear them off? With these antibacterial hand wipes, you can clear off the handle of the shopping basket and then feel great to take it and do your shopping for food. We can't see the germs that are surrounding us. Luckily with the handy moist disposable clothes, we don't have to see them by any stretch of the imagination. Wipe down the surface and go on about your business.

At the point when you eat in a hurry

Getting cheap food is some other time that you may need these hand wipes around. Once in a while, the drive-through doesn't give you napkins or gives you one when you need three. It is disappointing to have something on your hands and no real way to clear them off. If you have these wipes in your glove compartment, at that point, you are set! Pull one of these out and clear off your mind. Hurl it taken care of and proceed onward to your next goal.

Regardless of when you end up requiring hand wipes, you will consistently be happy that you had the prescience to place them in your handbag, in your pocket or your vehicle. They are flexible and can be used to clear off hands, faces and even surfaces, possibly your controlling wheel or that cup holder where the beverage overflowed. You won't need to stress over these little spills or clingy messes any longer, because you are set up to deal with them immediately. The wrecks that used to become bad dreams to tidy up never again occur - you are there with your hand wipes to ensure that.

At the point when the children need their hands cleaned because of the finger nourishments at the café or because of the soil in the play area, you are prepared. You don't need to attempt to dismiss the soil their hands or wipe off the clingy nectar mustard sauce with a dry napkin. You have moved past the wreckage. Clingy fingers are never again an issue; you have your hand wipes primed and ready. Sufficiently wet to handle the problem and permits their fingers to dry rapidly.

Hand Sanitizers for Effective Cleansing

Utilizing hand cleaning sanitizers is one of the most sterile methods for forestalling the simple spread of microorganisms. These items profess to slaughter 99.99% of the organisms present on the hand surfaces. The ethyl alcohol present in these sanitizers is profoundly successful in wrecking the microorganisms. They additionally accompany unique added substances to saturate your hands, leaving them delicate and revived. Hand sanitizers are accessible in compartments of fluctuating limits. For example, they come in 8 Oz siphon bottles, 1200 ml bottles, and so on.

Sanitizing Wipes - Convenient while on the Move

Washing hands with soap and water may not be conceivable when you are moving. This is the place sanitizing wipes prove to be useful. Stocking some in your sacks or pocket would be extremely useful when you are voyaging. Hand sanitizers are accessible in an assortment of arrangements, including gel, foam, and liquid mechanisms. They are pre-soaked wipes containing a lot of compelling chemicals. Oil, oil or any earth can be successfully expelled utilizing sanitizing wipes.

The fragile surfaces of these wipes help in exhaustive and compelling cleaning. To forestall sensitivities to the skin, they contain lanolin, aloe skin conditioners and gentle chemicals. This fabric like sanitizing wipes by and large accompany non-grating properties. Prevalent quality and non-abrasiveness are their additional highlights.

Do hand Sanitizing Wipes Kill Enough Germs fir them to be useful?

If you genuinely care about your cleanliness and sanitation, stocking the necessary number of hand cleaning sanitizers and sanitizing wipes is essential.

You might be comfortable with hand sanitizers in jugs or divider allocators. Hand sanitizing wipes can be an option for when these items are not accessible. You may be thinking about whether they are, for the most part, as compelling as the notices guarantee.

Hand sanitizing wipes eliminate germs for most purposes. As wipes are almost 100% compelling, you can use them to evacuate essential buildup on your hands, and consistently be guaranteed that they are perfect. Their germ-executing specialists are additionally useful in keeping microorganisms from spreading.

The principal advantage of this sort of sanitizer is that they are convenient. Regardless of whether you are voyaging or accomplishing open-air work or play, you don't have to search for a bathroom to clean your hands. They can be taken to work, or eateries, so it is anything but difficult to be sure about not contracting conceivably destructive germs from others.

A subsequent advantage regularly makes them ideal over distributors and containers. At the point when you use a wipe, you don't interact with microbes, which could have been left outwardly of the jug or container. Contains will, in general, be picked and put down, and distributors are regularly contacted and balanced. Neither of these issues happens with wipes. All you will ever have is the freshness you get from the wipes. Indeed, even open bathrooms won't be troublesome if you convey an inventory of wipes with you any place you go.

As they are expendable, it is both sterile and straightforward to discard used wipes. While most are not intended to be flushed down a toilet, they can be strategically located in a trash can or wastebasket. They don't have a cruel aroma, and some contain a unique scent, so they will be as charming to discard as they will be to use.

Nowadays, mainly, germs and microorganisms are a worry to everybody. From essential neatness to not having any desire to agreement or spread disease, great wellbeing is at the highest point of everybody's need list. Water won't be spotless your hands, and plain soap doesn't achieve significantly more. Picking a strategy that sterilizes every single time advances better wellbeing for yourself and others around you.

At the point when you select a hand sanitizing wipe, with or without an additional aroma, keeping your hands clean and sans germ is pure. Whenever of the day or night, eating, working, and playing will all be more beneficial.

Reasons why you ought to consistently keep Wipes Handy

Hand wipes: they are likely not something that you would consider in most passing discussions, with a particular case to perhaps an occurrence where you just got your hands all slimy and require them. While the appearance and ubiquity of hand sanitizing items are turning out to be increasingly typical (hell, some supermarkets much offer containers out front so you can disinfect your shopping basket handles), hand wipes are likewise a choice. For the most part, they can fill in as preferable alternatives over merely depending upon hand sanitizer. What follows are the top reasons why it bodes well to consistently keep some hand wipes, well, handy during your everyday undertakings.

1. It's a grimy world where we live and that restroom sink and inviting container of antibacterial soap are not in every case close enough for comfort.

2. Do you contact cash every day? Did you realize that money is the dirtiest thing on the planet that you can touch because such a significant number of individuals are continually contacting it? With hand wipes, you can clean the green after you delicate installment.

3. So you needed to use the bathroom critically and it is necessary that you made a stopover at a spot that you typically could never visit. After hunching down to guarantee that your wellbeing is protected in the bathroom, you out of nowhere acknowledge after attempting to wash your hands that there is no soap and its hand wipes to save by and by.

4. Did you, at any point, go on an excursion? Numerous parks don't highlight washrooms nowadays. A paper towel or napkin can help. In any case, shouldn't something be said about getting the grime off your mind and sanitizing them when you eat?

5. Accomplish your work out at the exercise center now and again? Most exercise center machines are unsanitary, regardless of whether they seem, by all accounts, to be perfect. Sweat-soaked individuals turning out in them like clockwork guarantees this measurement. In any case, you can without much of a stretch exercise and inhale pure by cleaning them down and sanitizing them beforehand.

6. Do you have youngsters going around? Children are a delight; however, they can, in general, get rather messy rather rapidly. Some handy hand wipes will destroy this stress from regularly concerning you.

7. The market is our entry to tasty culinary eats. It can likewise be the door to you becoming ill. So be sure to wipe down those shopping basket handles and execute any germs on them before contacting them with your hands.

8. So you don't use paper cash because it is squalid. Great call, money is exceptionally gross when you truly consider what number of hands it crosses. However, prepare to be blown away. That charge pin machine at the store finds to be many germ loaded fingers contacting it, as well. So wipe it down genuine snappy before touching it.

9. Made a wreck unintentionally? You will miss those hand wipes when you need them the most.

10. Need a simple method to disinfect things? Hand wipes are smaller and fit in many pockets and comfortably into most wallets.

Sterile Wipes-Undervalued and Underappreciated in Households?

Sterile wipes are a typical household sanitation item that is regularly overlooked and underestimated. Be that as it may, in truth, it is a significant item to individuals, particularly with relatives. Disinfectant wipes execute off germs and microscopic organisms from hands, feet, face, and in any piece of the body. It diminishes the danger of contaminations and spreading germs. It is one of the family's best apparatuses for wellbeing anticipation.

The disorder is so widespread nowadays. Viruses and bugs are transforming too rapidly that the clinical research groups are making some hard memories keeping up, in case stay in front of the perils. Influenza shots are currently rendered useless and have gotten deadly sometimes. This makes it increasingly down to earth to keep your family protected against illnesses and contaminations.

What's more, it will be commonsense to show your children the significance of sterile wipes right off the bat. Wipes have been demonstrated to viably diminish, slow down and kill the spread of unsafe viruses and microscopic organisms. So make sure to keep them in washrooms, kitchens, rooms, in your vehicle, in your handbag, your kids' knapsacks, and anyplace you can consider.

Microbes can be executed off by sanitizers, gels and water, however insufficient to evacuate additional hints of soil and grime. Additionally, there are heavier to heft around because of their containers. Wipes, then again, are handier. You can clear your hands to keep off from soil when dinners. It is likewise imperative to wash hands after managing exercises that may move microbes to your hands. For example, cleaning out your nose, hacking, contacting creatures, handling cash, opening door handles, driving, playing outside, shaking hands and utilizing the restroom. The microbes flourish in cold and clammy zones, for example, on handles and restrooms, so always remember to disinfect hands at whatever point they need emerges.

Wipes are likewise used in numerous business territories, for example, out in the open restrooms, accommodation stores, clinical centers, dental centers, emergency clinics and other clinical offices. The clinical field has observed the significance of antibacterial wipes to dispose of germs.

Antibacterial wipes are additionally called wet disposable clothes, for they are soaked with Chlorohexidine Gluconate or Isopropyl Alcohol, or both. Wipes come in all shapes, amounts and estimates, and different brands to browse available. They are additionally accessible in mixed bundling to make them fit for each sort of circumstance.

Germs are all over, so it is sheltered to consistently keep clean wipes at close reach, much the same as a medical aid unit. Never venture out from home for work, school or family trip without germicide wipes. There is no constrained measure of wipes to use at some random time-you can use it as frequently and the same number of times as you need. By playing it safe and keeping your hands clean, you will have the option to forestall maladies like hepatitis, salmonella, influenza, hacks and flu.

Antibacterial Wipes or Disinfectant Wipes, which to use?

Many individuals don't know about the contrasts between items with antibacterial properties and those that are disinfectants. It is an important distinction as the use of wet disposable clothes, gels and sanitizing hand wipes has detonated as of late. Despite the fact that the use of these items has unequivocally been prescribed to control the spread of viruses and lessen the pace of bacterial infections, for any situation, it is essential to know the distinctions.

For the most part, antibacterial wipes are used on hands to eliminate microscopic organisms and forestall its transmission. Liquid hand sanitizers will execute these germs too; however, they won't expel hints of nourishment, soil and grime. Gels, despite everything, have their place as these little jugs can be put pretty much anywhere, and they are a very financially savvy technique for controlling the transmission of ailment. The preponderance of nut sensitivities today demands that schools depend upon antibacterial wipes after dinners and tidbits. It is favored that hand wipes are evaluated "Non-Hazardous" and contain a hand protecting oil.

It is a typical confusion that dishwashing fluids, likewise claiming to be antibacterial hand cleansers, will be compelling on household surfaces, for example, cutting sheets, appliance handles, and ledges. The cleaning procedure for hands versus hardware varies significantly. With hands, we will, in general, scour and rub our hands together, which incredibly helps the cleaning procedure. With equipment, we will clear it off. Consequently, a more successful technique is to use disinfectant wipes on surfaces.

Disinfecting wipes by differentiating are commonly used on shared office machines, seats, exercise center hardware, shopping trucks or in the kitchen and restrooms. They are powerful on many viruses just as microscopic organisms. Often alcohol is the active ingredient in disinfectants. Alcohol is profoundly combustible and evaporates rapidly. You should drench the item to obtain compelling disinfection. Chlorine dye is another choice. However, it is very scathing to the skin, lungs and eyes. And, erroneously combining it with alkali or any other acid, for example, vinegar brings about the creation of harmful gas. Since there are smelling salts in the urine, use around pets and in restrooms can be dangerous also that both are very stinking. Thus, water-based engineered phenolic mixes are significantly liked.

Many marvels, whether custom made mixtures are powerful. Studies have exhibited that the more significant part of these has practically no disinfectant properties. When dealing with a particular disease, for example, hepatitis, influenza, salmonella, and so on, you should use the best yet safe substance and methods accessible. Thoroughly washing and drying hands and surfaces alongside the use of antibacterial wipes and disinfecting wipes is the best counteraction you will find.

Baby Wipes

Baby wipes are dispensable materials used to cleanse the touchy skin of infants. These materials are produced using non-woven textures like those used in dryer sheets and are soaked with an answer of delicate cleansing ingredients. Baby wipes are generally sold in plastic tubs that keep the fabrics soggy and consider simple dispensing.

Are Baby Wipes Antibacterial?

In almost all cases, baby wipes are not antibacterial because the alcohol or sanitizing synthetic concoctions would be excessively irritating to a baby's skin. Fortunately, baby wipes shouldn't be antibacterial because it isn't essential to keep your baby safe and clean. Ordinary showers with foamy water are the best arrangement.

There is a lot of approaches to keep your baby clean, and it would bode well that antibacterial wipes may be something to be thankful for to have when cleaning up your baby and her wrecks. We should plunge into why most baby wipes aren't antibacterial and look at the best ones to use to keep your baby's base feeling acceptable.

Think about the last time you went through the day cleaning up your house without gloves on or used an excessive amount of hand sanitizer. Your hands were most likely feeling somewhat like sandpaper before the day's over, and you were running for some moisturizer.

Since a baby's skin isn't as intense as an adult's, a lot of synthetic compounds and even alcohol based sanitizers can be very drying and irritating for infants and babies. On the off chance that you consider the way that infants will have their diaper changed about multiple times every day, combined with a few hand and face wipes, it's not hard to imagine your baby's skin getting red and bothered.

While it's easy to think that you ought to be continually sanitizing a baby's bottom after filthy diapers, a tad of baby crap is profoundly improbable to cause issues like diaper rash or infections except if the dirty diaper is left on for a significant period or there are cuts or other open injuries here. Try not to misunderstand me; it's still gross. You simply don't need to bleach the baby's bottom each opportunity something turns out.

Under normal circumstances, your baby will be okay.

If you ever observe redness, disturbance, sores, rashes, or anything else strange, then you ought to presumably think about an outing to the pediatrician. While most bothering will leave all alone, yeasty rashes will, as a rule, require an antifungal.

What are the most well-known sanitizing synthetic compounds in antibacterial wipes?

By a wide margin, the most well-known kind of concoction that you'll find in a run of the mill antibacterial wipe is what's known as a quat (quaternary ammonium compound), and they will appear under many changed names. If you are checking marks, search for any of these:

- Didecyl dimethyl ammonium chloride

- Dioctyl dimethyl ammonium chloride

- Alkyl dimethyl benzyl ammonium chloride

- Alkyl dimethyl ethyl benzyl ammonium chloride

- Benzalkonium chloride

- Benzethonium chloride

The beneficial thing about these synthetic substances is that they have been demonstrated to execute many dangerous microorganisms, for example, E. coli and Staph, when used as suggested. The issue is that they are unreasonably stable for most household needs in the fixations found in antibacterial showers and wipes and too solid to even think about cleaning up human skin, particularly pampers!

Quats are known irritants to the lungs, particularly for those with sensitivities and asthma. They are additionally known skin irritants and can create rashes if you leave them on the skin excessively long, or the focus is too high. Fun truth, most antibacterial wipes will advise you to wash your hands after use which invalidates the point of using them to clean up in any case

Alcohol-based wipes and sanitizers can be used in a pinch.

You don't generally approach a bath, so there are circumstances in which antibacterial wipes or sanitizers can be useful. If you are out and about or in any case out on the town, you should have a couple of handy in the event of some unforeseen issue.

The CDC suggests using wipes or sanitizers that contain synthetic substances like the quats we discussed before. Instead, they prescribe a alcohol based sanitizer or wipe that has in any event 60 percent alcohol in the mix. This fixation has been demonstrated to rapidly drop the number of dangerous microorganisms on your hands under perfect circumstances. It won't cause a lot of disturbance as the quats because they quickly evaporate into the air instead of sticking around.

Making Your Sanitizing Wipes Using Different Recipes

In case you're worried about getting debilitated during the coronavirus flare-up, chances are you're taking the entirety of the essential strides to remain sound (washing your hands, not touching your face, wiping down much of the time used surfaces, and so on.). Be that as it may, one issue many individuals have experienced during this time is fundamental cleaning supplies being sold out wherever because of popular demand. Instead of searching far and wide for costly cleaning wipes, did you realize you can make your own for not exactly a dollar? With vinegar and fluid dish cleanser, you'll love the excellent way this simple DIY can be made again and again with the assistance of a repurposed coffee canister. Produced using every natural ingredient, you can even include a couple of sprinkles of your favorite essential oil to customize these eco-accommodating cleaning wipes.

What You'll Need

- One-pound coffee canister with plastic cover
- Paper towel roll
- Sharp blade
- 1/2 cup vinegar
- 1/4 cup water
- 1/4 cup rubbing liquor
- 1 teaspoon fluid dish cleanser
- 10 drops fundamental oil (discretionary)
- Spray paint (discretionary)
- Needle
- Scissors

Directions:

- The ingredients for these custom made wipes cost pretty much nothing, which means you can have a can of wipes in each room of your home. Vinegar works admirably of cleaning while normally whisking germs ceaselessly, preventing mold, and killing microscopic organisms. And you can use your favorite dish cleanser or make your own.

- Repurposing an old coffee can for this DIY makes a container or vessel that can be used again and again. Either leave the box as it is or give it an active layer of shower paint, inside and out, for a new look and to keep the inside of the can from rusting.

- To make the cleaning wipes, cut the paper towels down the middle using a sharp serrated blade, and squish them into the painted can. And using eco-accommodating paper towels makes this DIY considerably greener.

- Mix the vinegar, dish cleanser, rubbing liquor, and water in a little bowl. You can include a few drops of fundamental oil to the wipes, which customizes the cleaner and lifts its antibacterial forces

- Slowly pour the fluid over the paper towels. When they're soaked, cautiously evacuate the cardboard place, and pull a paper towel from the center.

- Press a specialty needle through the focal point of the plastic top a few times, and then fit the scissors through to cut a hover from the inside, around one half-inch in the distance across.

- Now feed the paper towel through the gap in the plastic cover and secure it to the painted coffee can (to keep the wipes soggy, include a couple of drops of water into the canister). Presently you have handcrafted wipes that are extraordinary at cleaning and disinfecting your home!

Disinfectant Wipes-Reusable Clorox Wipes

The extraordinary thing about disinfecting wipes is that you realize you are getting something clean when you use them. Roughly 99% of the germs are no more. The terrible thing about those equivalent wipes is that they can cost a considerable lot, and they are going to our landfill because they can't be reused. They have a spot and a reason for sure. In any case, if you want to figure out how to make disinfectant wipes that can be washed and reused, at that point, you will adore this formula for REUSABLE DIY Clorox Wipes!

Ingredients:

- 3 cups of refined water

- ¾ cup of rubbing liquor

- 6 teaspoon of Dawn dishwashing cleanser (change the sum to suit)

- 10 drops of Lemon Essential Oil

- 10 Washcloths

- Glass container

"You could use either tap water or filtered water in your natively constructed cleaning items. The explanations behind using refined versus faucet water would rely upon your nearby faucet water. On the off chance that your faucet water has a ton of minerals in it (for example on the off chance that you have hard water), it could leave "watermarks", which would be annoying when you're trying to clean!"

Instructions:

- First, choose how huge you want your wipes. I cut the vast majority of my washcloths down the middle, yet I left some full size for bigger occupations.

- Fill your container with the washcloths.

- In a bowl, mix water, rubbing liquor, Dawn and lemon fundamental oil

- Pour the cleaning mix into the container over the washcloths.

- Put the cover on and use varying. After your clothes are messy, toss in the washing machine and redo as essential.

Making Sanitizing Wipes Using Essential Oils (Lemon and Lavender)

Accumulate collapsed baby wipes or divided napkins in a container with a top.

Mix:

- $1^{1}/_{2}$ ^{c} warm water

- 1 tablespoon of coconut oil

- 1 teaspoon of rubbing alcohol or vodka

- 3 drops of Lavender essential oil

- 3 drops of Lemon essential oil

Ensure the coconut has liquefied into the water at that point pour the mixture onto the stack(s) of wipes. On the off chance that you are using the baby wipes, you won't need to use the total of the liquid.

Making Disinfectant Wipes with Coconut oil, Witch Hazel and Lavender

These wipes use a ton of indistinguishable ingredients from the hand sanitizer. The lavender oil in this formula is antiseptic while additionally soothing for the skin, making it perfect for wipes used on the surface.

Materials

- Paper towels or napkins
- Container with cover
- 1 cup of water
- 1 Tablespoon of coconut oil
- ¼ cup witch hazel
- 8 drops lavender fundamental oil

Instructions

Heat some water on the stove, allowing it to cool to a warm temperature before mixing it with different ingredients. While you set up the water, overlay the paper towels or napkins, so they fit cozily in your container. When the water is only a warm temperature, mix the coconut oil into it until the oil has softened totally and scattered all through the water. Mix in the witch hazel and lavender essential oil. Pour the fluid over the wipes in the container, soaking every one of them. Put the cover on the box and use the wipes varying.

I hope this book provides you with all the knowledge and information required to making your Sanitizers, Soaps and Wipes.

Thank you for your time!

www.ingramcontent.com/pod-product-compliance
Lightning Source LLC
Chambersburg PA
CBHW071407210526
45465CB00001B/292